COLORS of HOPE

Breast Cancer Warriors Coloring Book
(Volume One)

by April McCallum

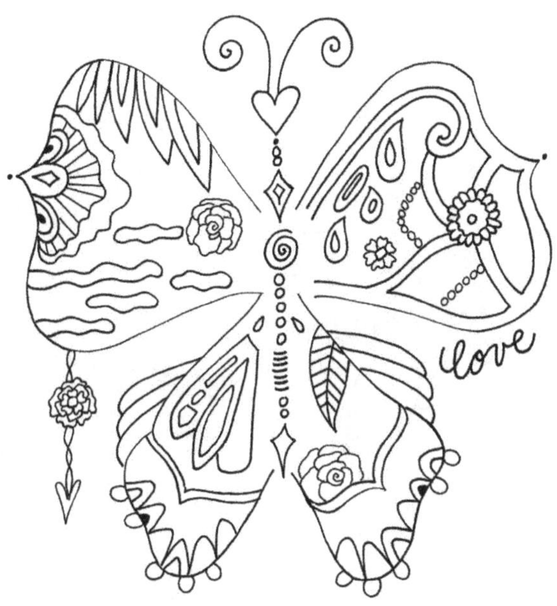

ISBN: 978-1-7325752-3-3

Colors of Hope: Breast Cancer Warriors Coloring Book Volume One
© 2018 by April McCallum
Published in the United States by Heart and Key Publishing

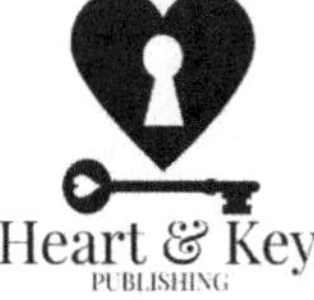

Cover Design Collaboration and Colorization by Pete Berg
www.aprilmccallumdesigns.com

Dedication

This book, *Colors of Hope*, is dedicated to my mother, aunt, mother-in-law and dear friends, along with all of the beautiful breast cancer warriors and survivors who've fought valiantly one day at a time. A special shout out to the researchers, funders and healthcare professionals who make it their mission to find a cure. So many of you say you are not brave because you didn't choose this, it chose you. But the rest of us cheering you on think you are, because you chose not to give up.

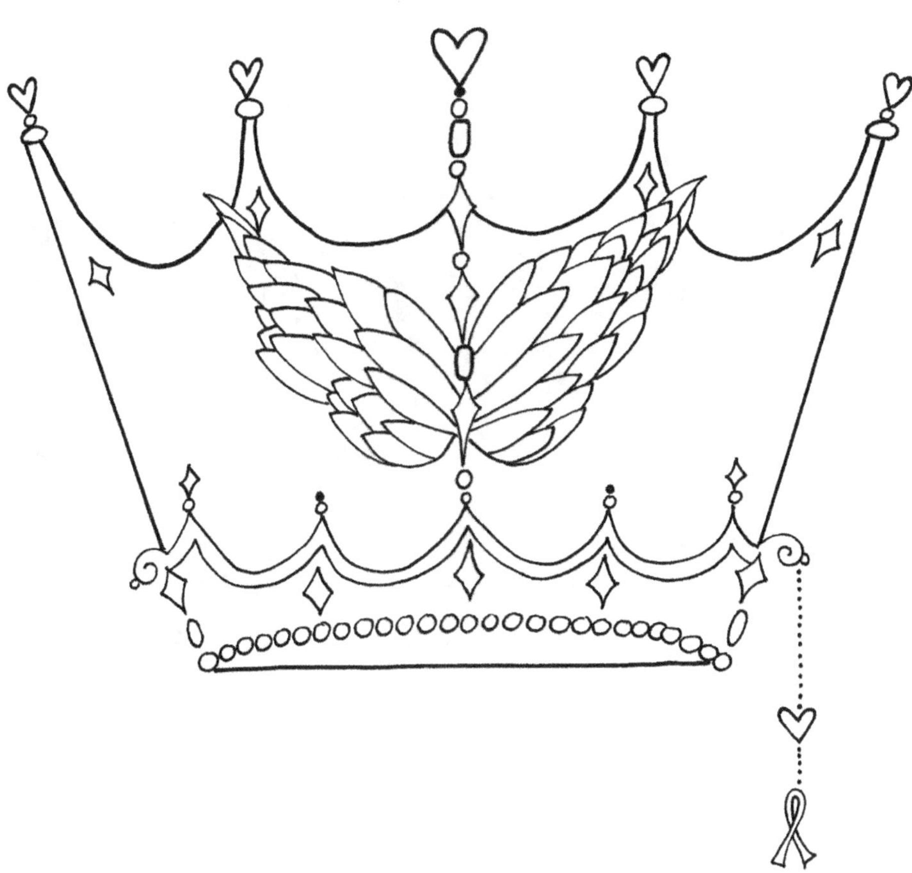

Welcome!

Art and Heart... I'm so happy you're here! I've created some hand-drawn coloring pages with love, just for you! Several years ago I began creating collections of advocacy art. My aunt, mother-in-law and a couple of dear friends battled breast cancer. I wanted to play some small part in raising awareness of this toxic disease that was touching so many women in such a personal way.

Little did I know that years later, my 80-plus-year-old mother would also become a breast cancer warrior. And warrior she was! Bless her brave little heart. Gratefully, she is now on the survivors list. But the battle continues for so many women *and men!* After an up-close-and-personal walk with my mother through a lumpectomy, chemotherapy and radiation treatments, I wanted to do more.

Colors of Hope was designed to give you a therapeutic coloring experience that will fill your mind and heart with strength and positivity. This collection of coloring pages was created to make colorists feel loved, filled with beauty, inspiration, hope and courage while going through treatments.

Tips: You will notice a bit of extra margin on the binding side. I intentionally designed it that way for ease of maneuvering. If you would like to practice your lines and coloring tools, you will find a blank page in the back of the book to do just that. If you plan to use non-dry coloring materials (like markers), please place a blank sheet or two under the page you're coloring so it doesn't bleed through. When it comes to art and therapeutic coloring, it's all about the heart. There is no right or wrong, good or bad. Consider this book a place for you "to go" to get lost in uplifting thoughts and color.

Thank you for allowing me to share just a little of my art and heart with you!

XO

April

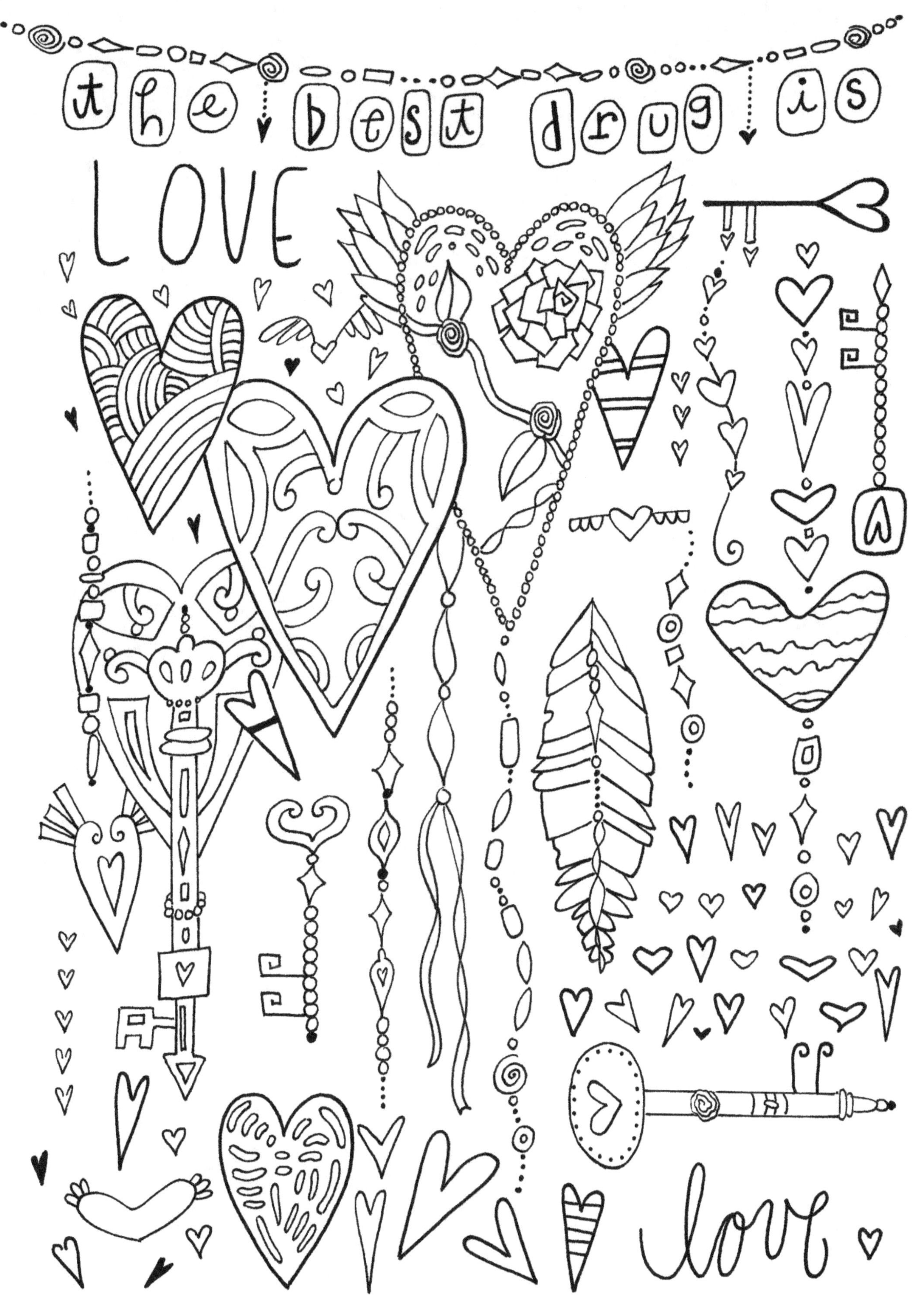
the best drug is
LOVE
love

HOPE
is stronger than
FEAR

Never have ♥ Never Will

My ⋗boobs⋖ do not
DEFINE ME.

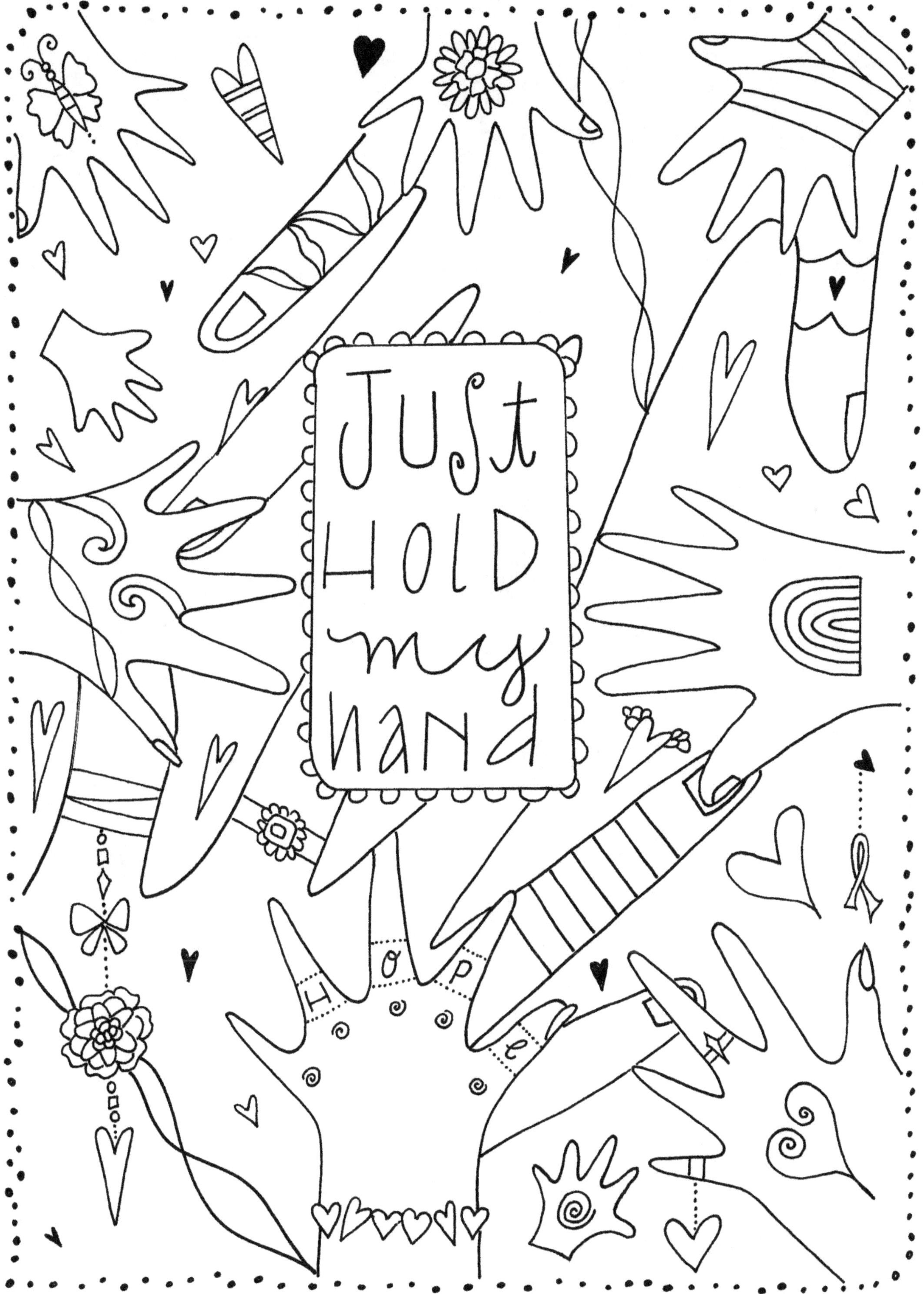

JUST
HOLD
my
hand
HOPE

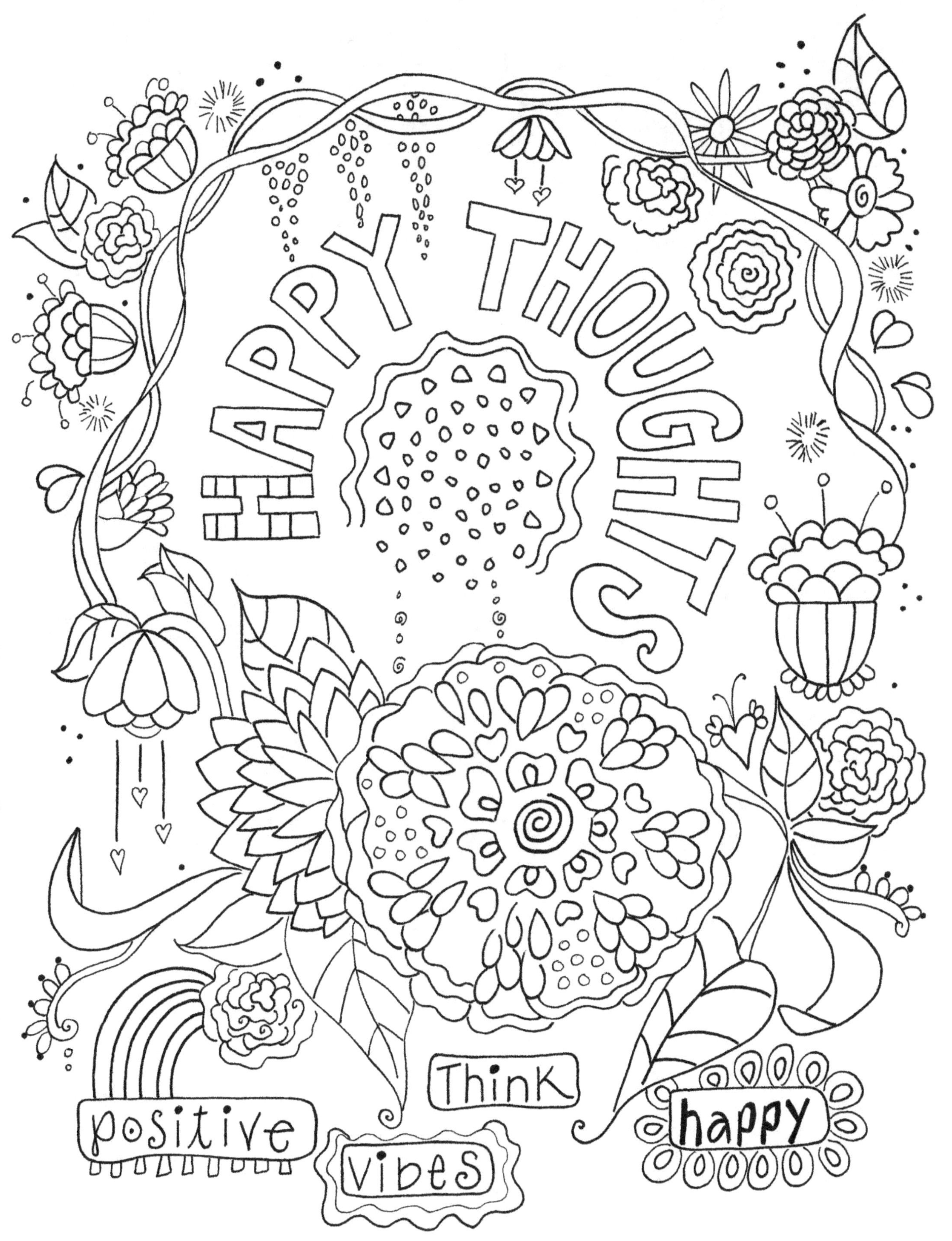

HAPPY THOUGHTS
positive
Think
vibes
happy

My Scarves, My Friends.

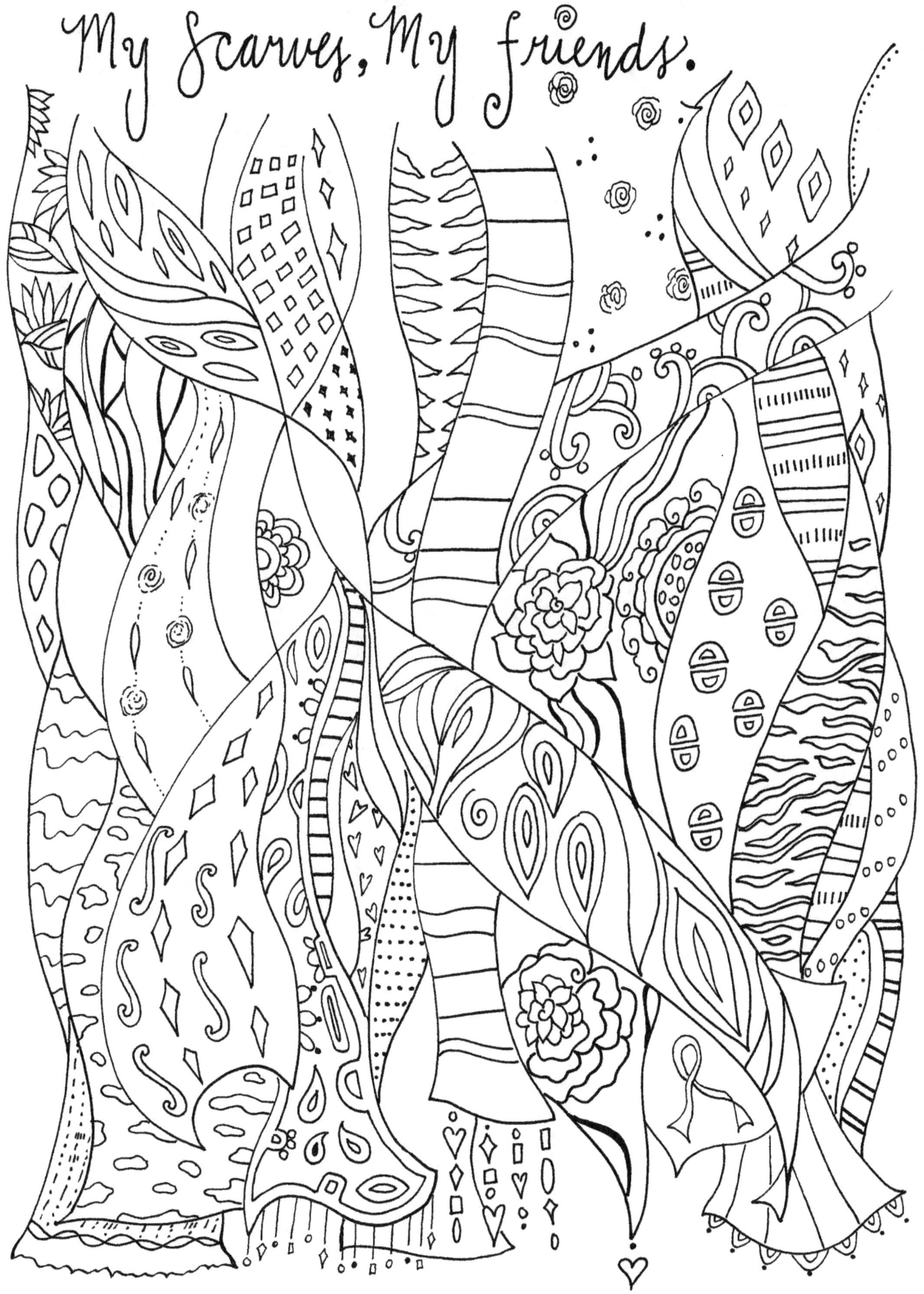

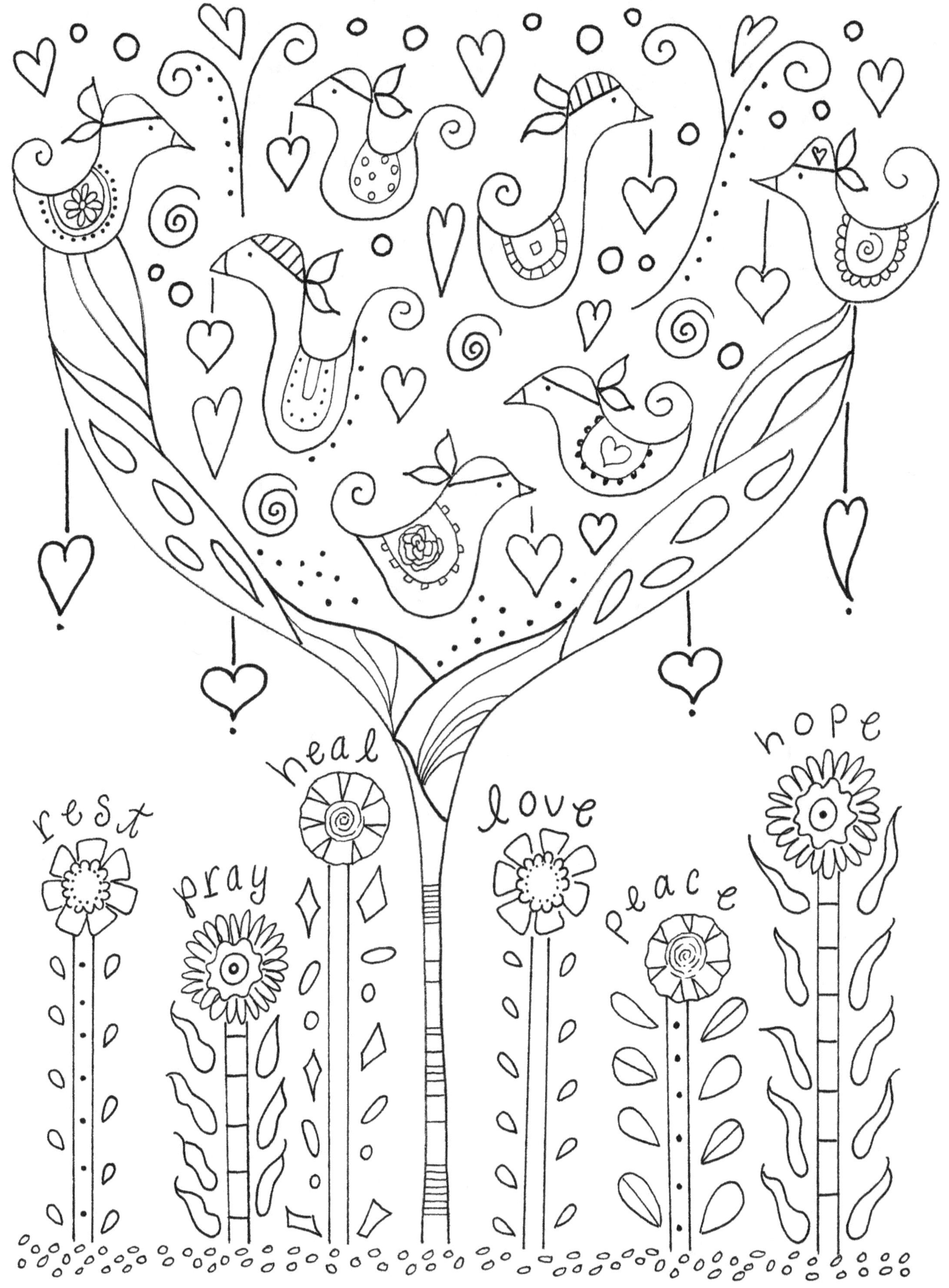

rest
pray
heal
love
peace
hope

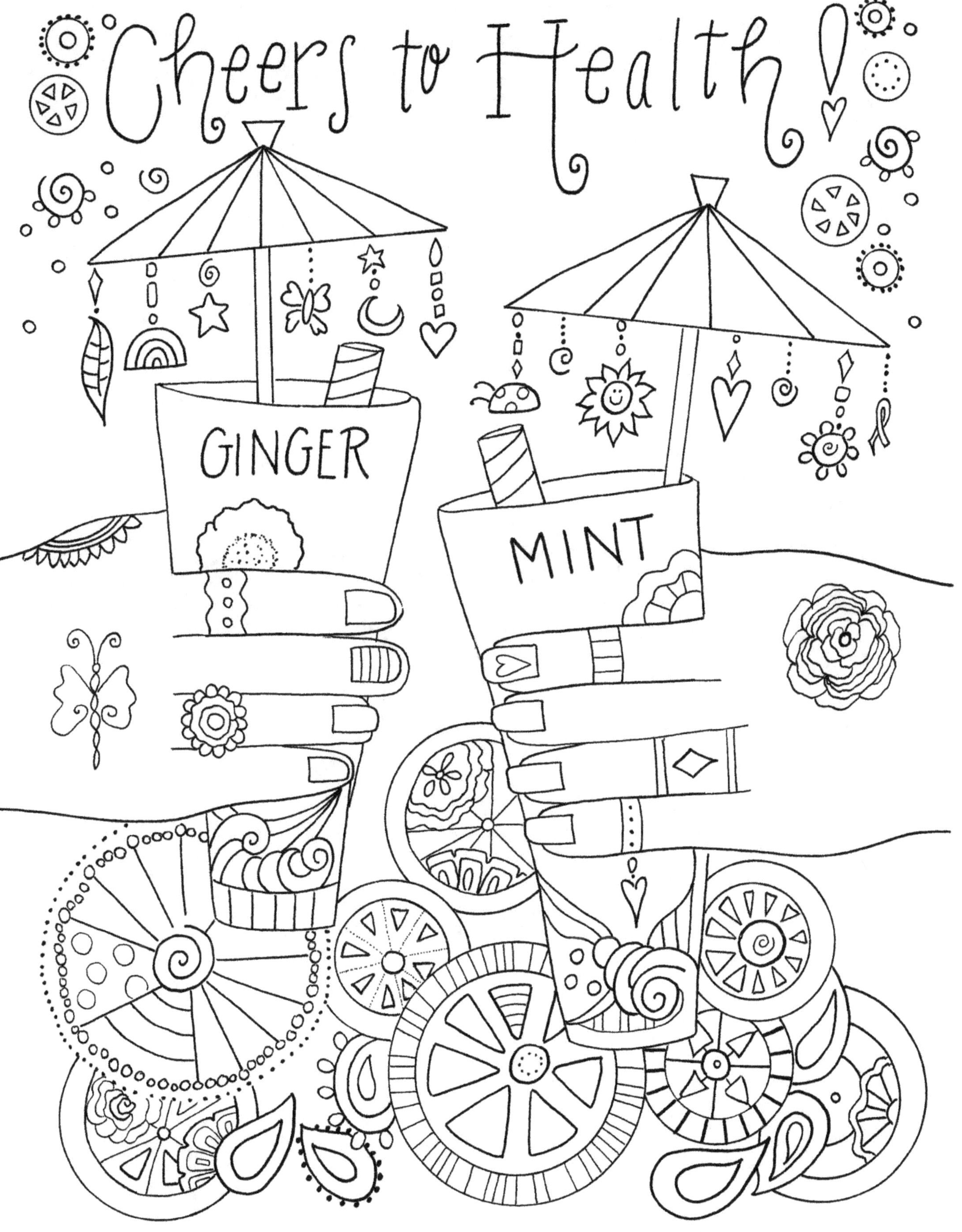

Cheers to Health!
GINGER
MINT

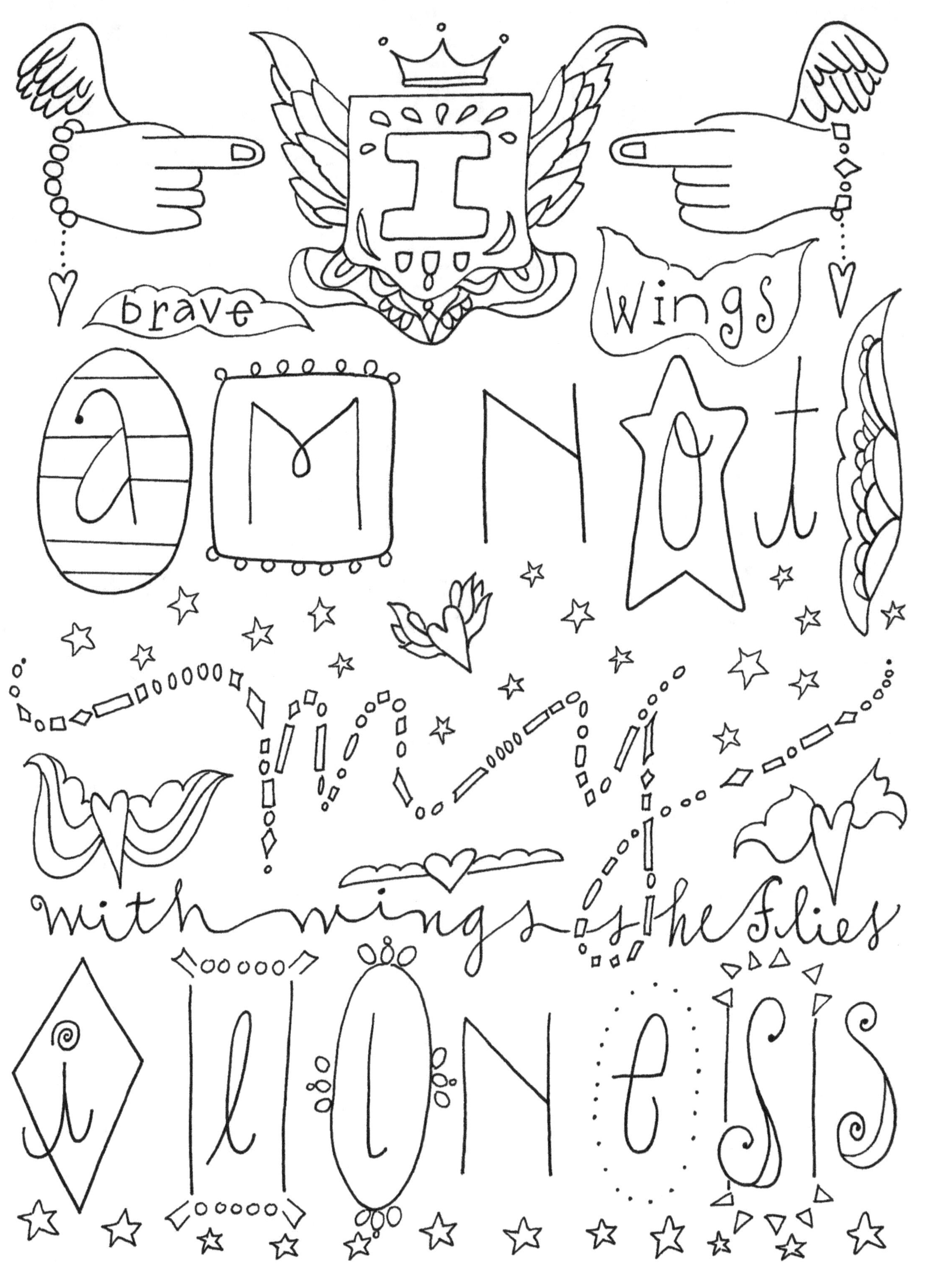

brave wings
I AM NOT
with wings she flies
I AM NOT ALONE IS

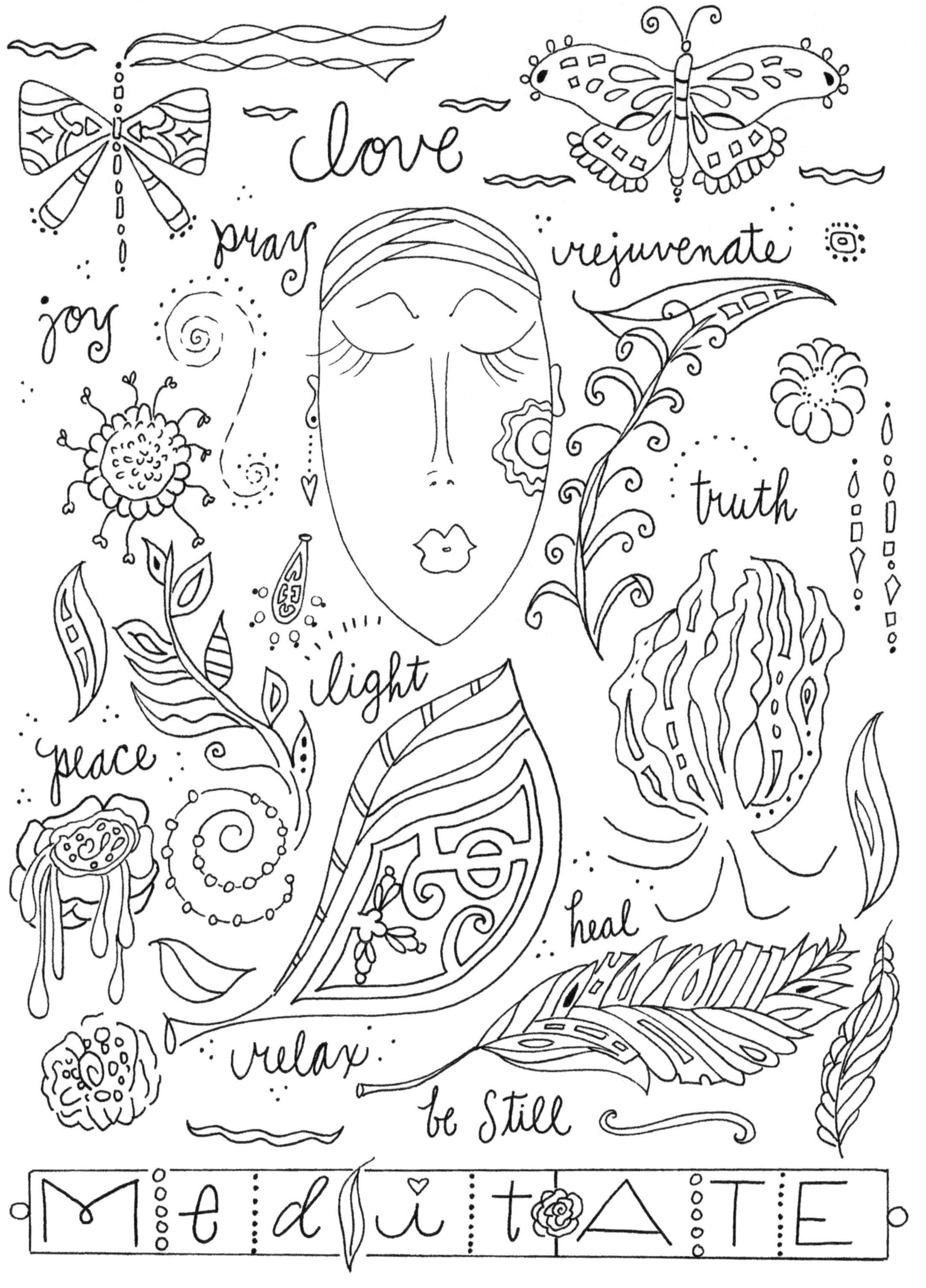

~love~
pray
rejuvenate
joy
truth
light
peace
heal
relax
be still
MEDITATE

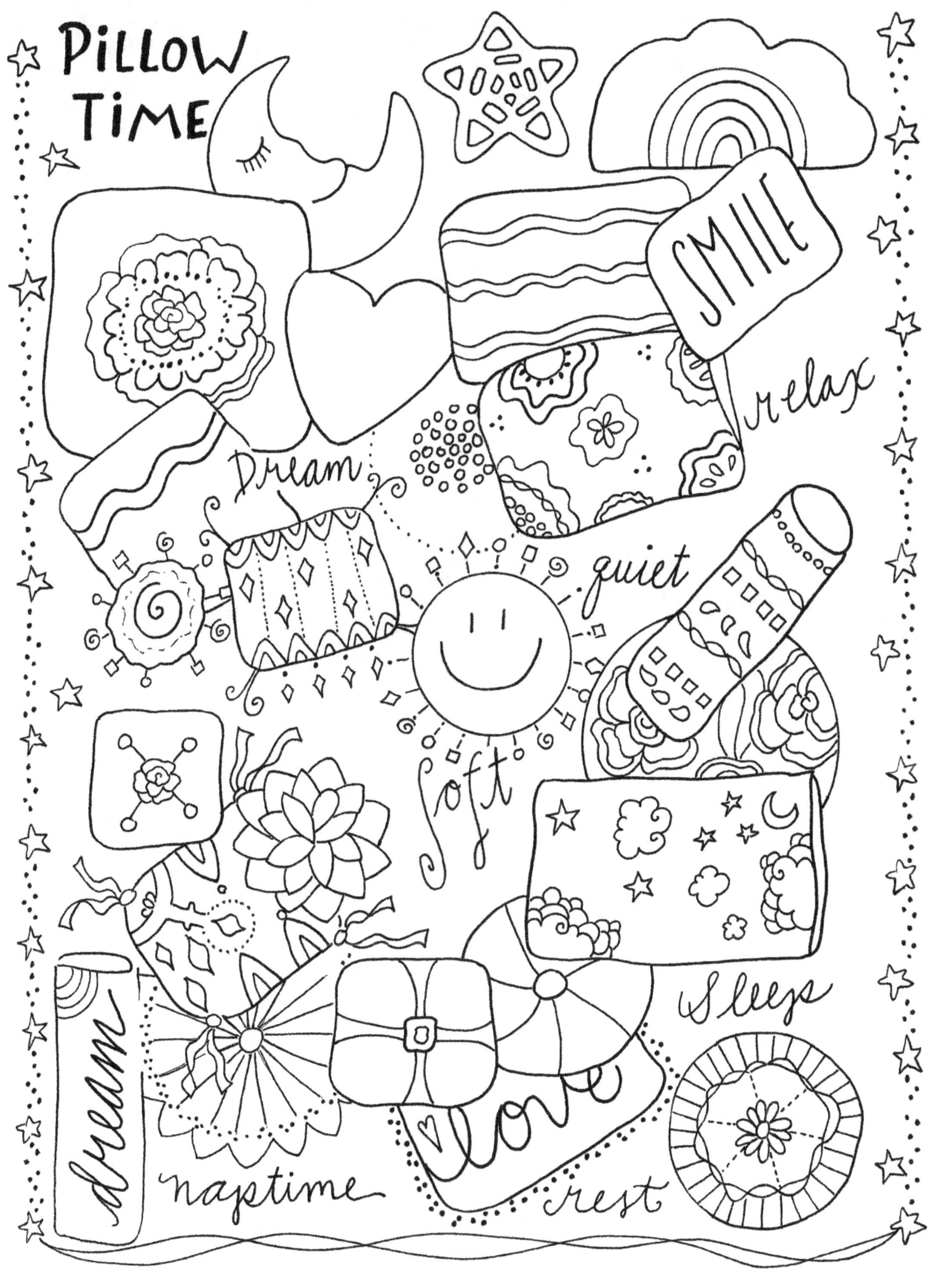

PiLLOW TIME
SMILE
relax
Dream
quiet
soft
Sleep
dream
naptime
love
rest

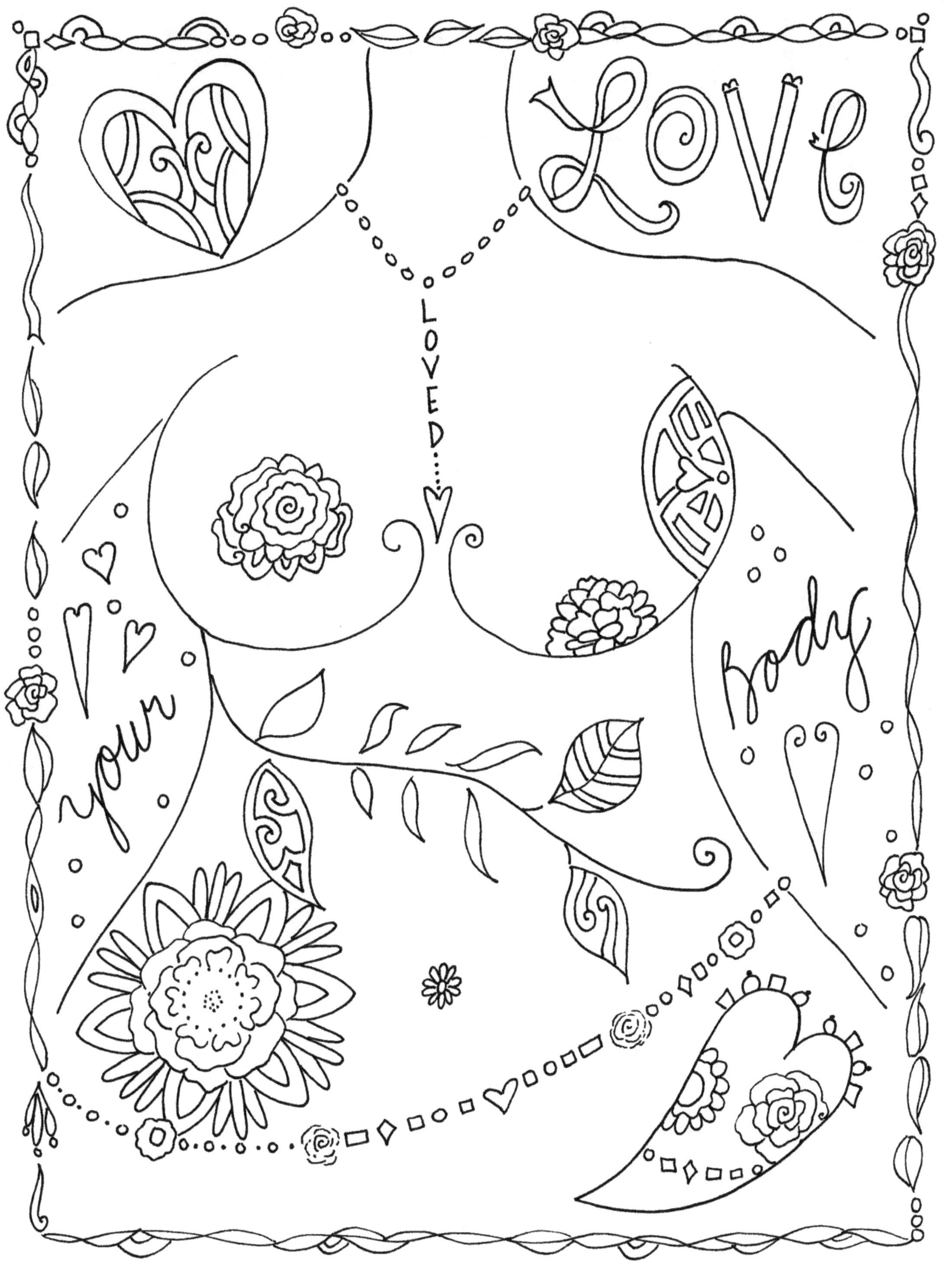
Love
LOVED
your
Body

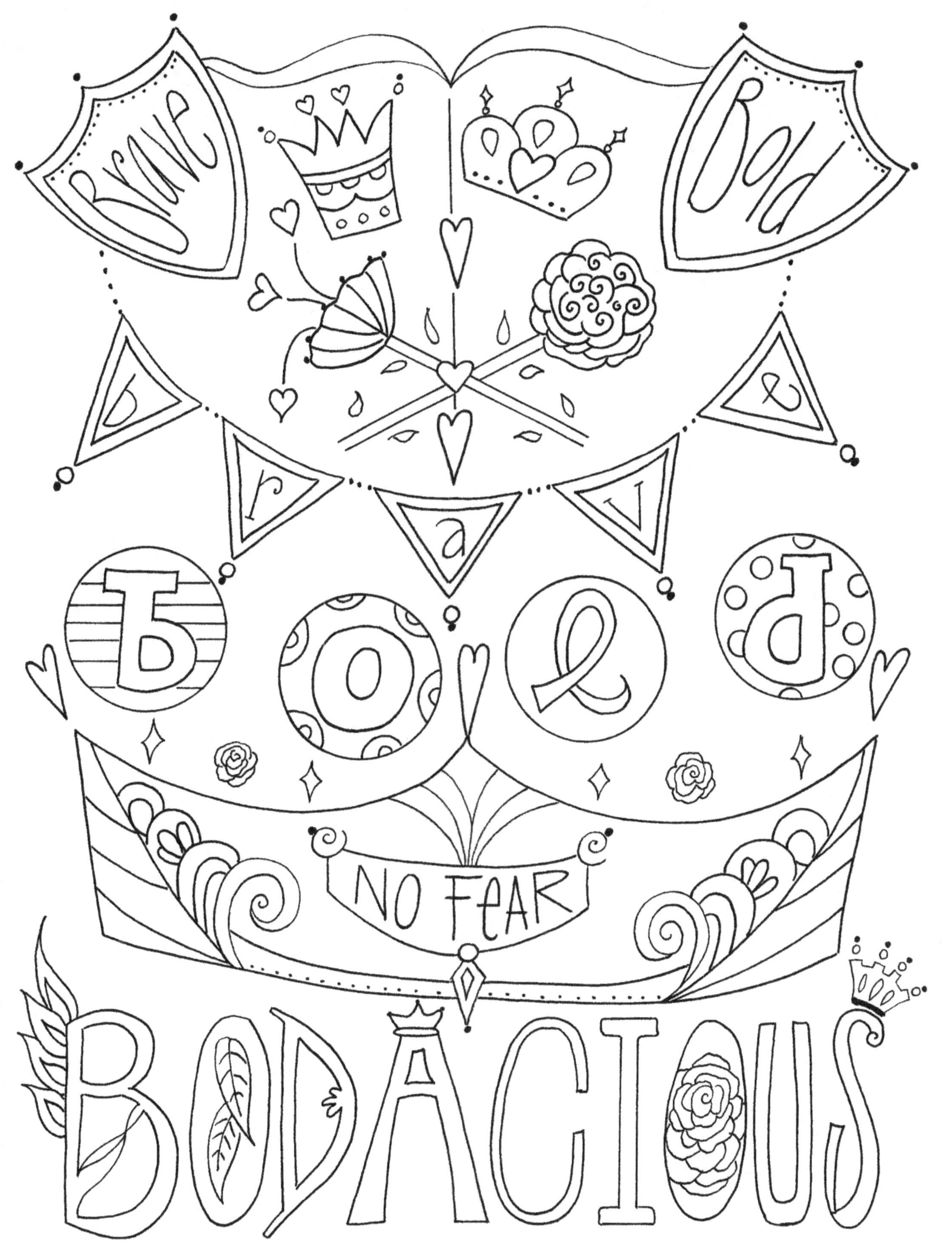

Brave
Bold
No Fear
BODACIOUS

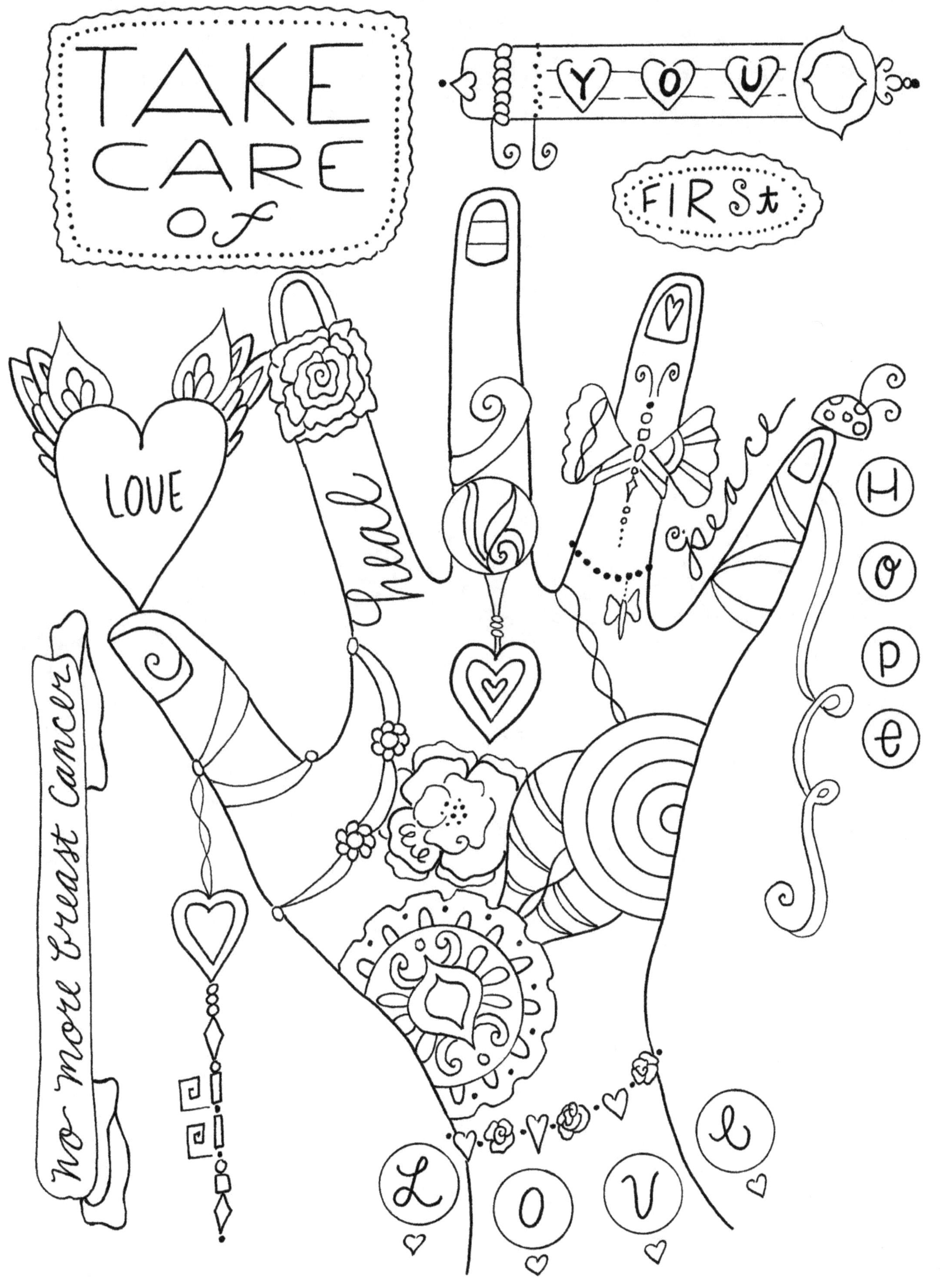

TAKE CARE of
YOU
FIRST
LOVE
heal
peace
HOPE
no more breast cancer
LOVE

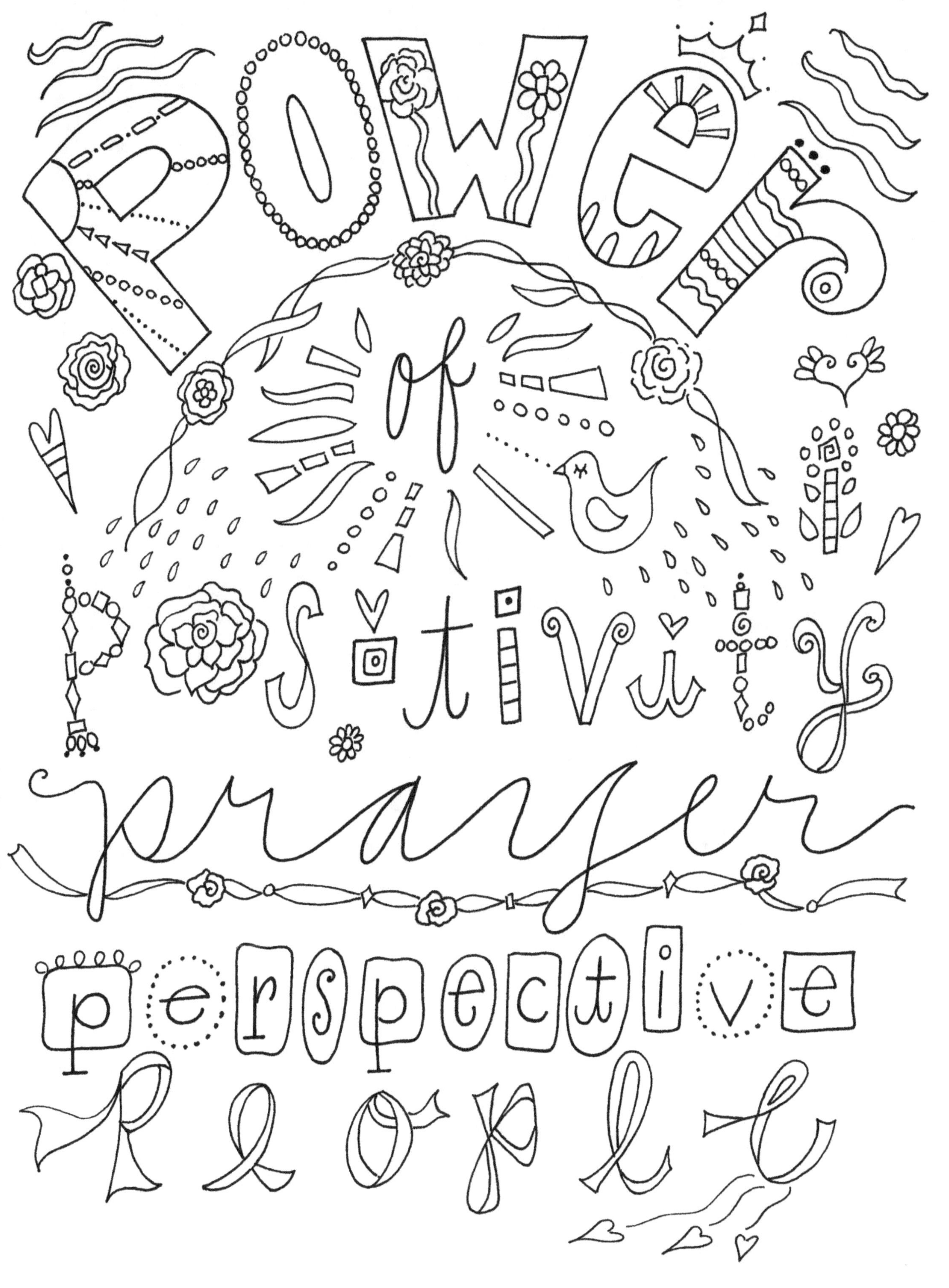

Power
of
Positivity
prayer
perspective
People

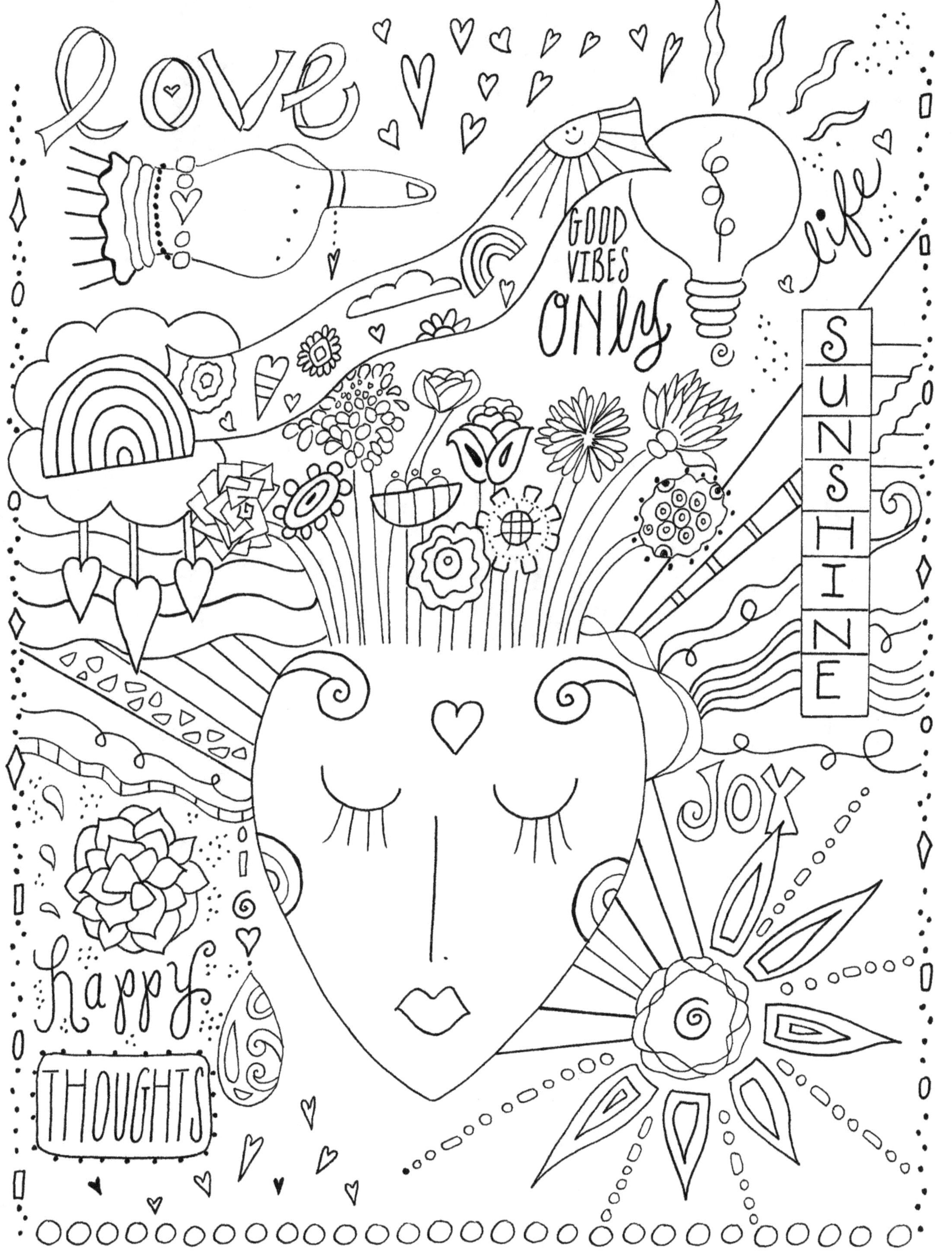

love
GOOD VIBES ONLY
life
SUNSHINE
JOY
happy
THOUGHTS

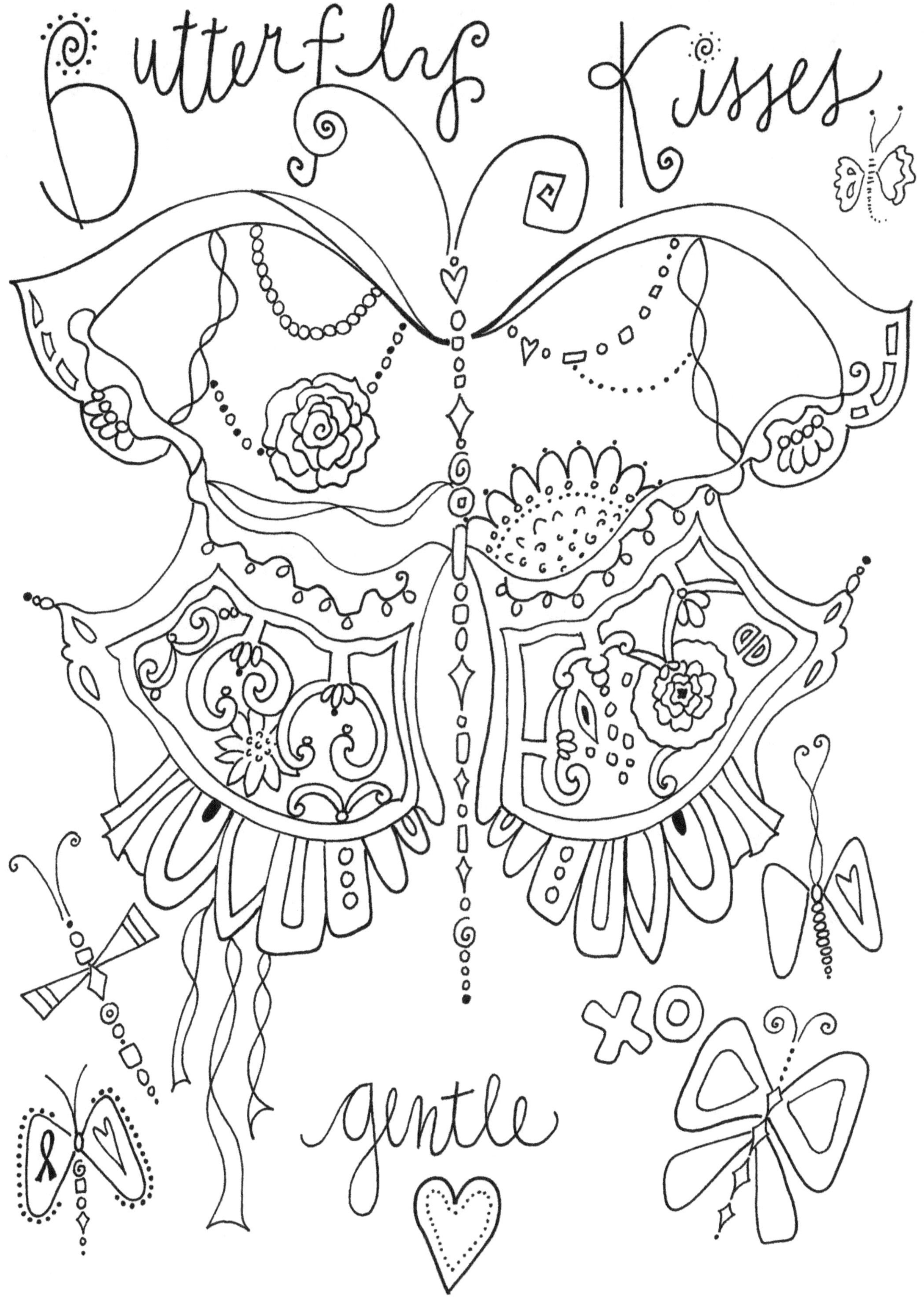

Butterfly Kisses
gentle
XO

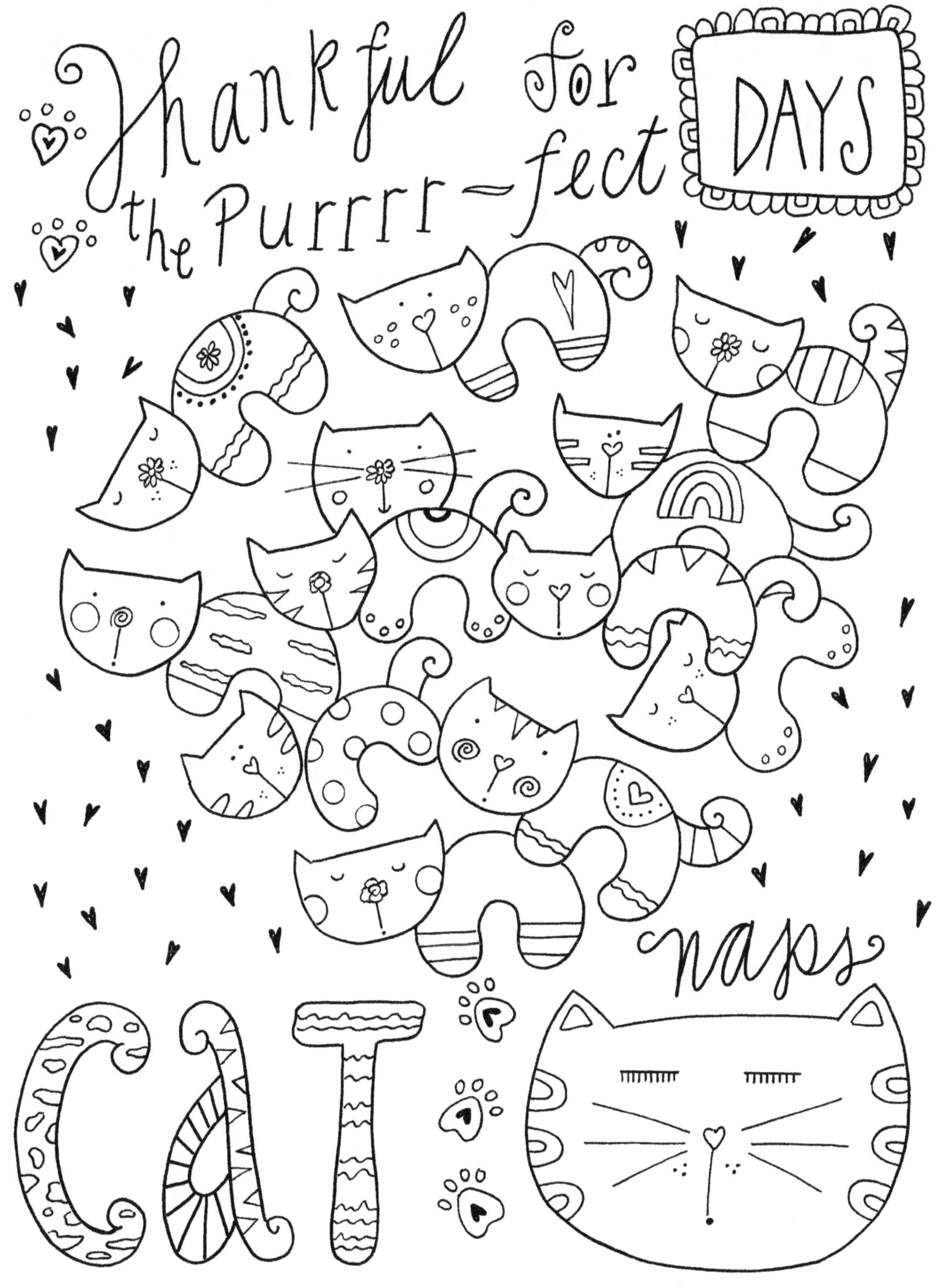

Thankful for
the Purrrr-fect DAYS
naps
CAT

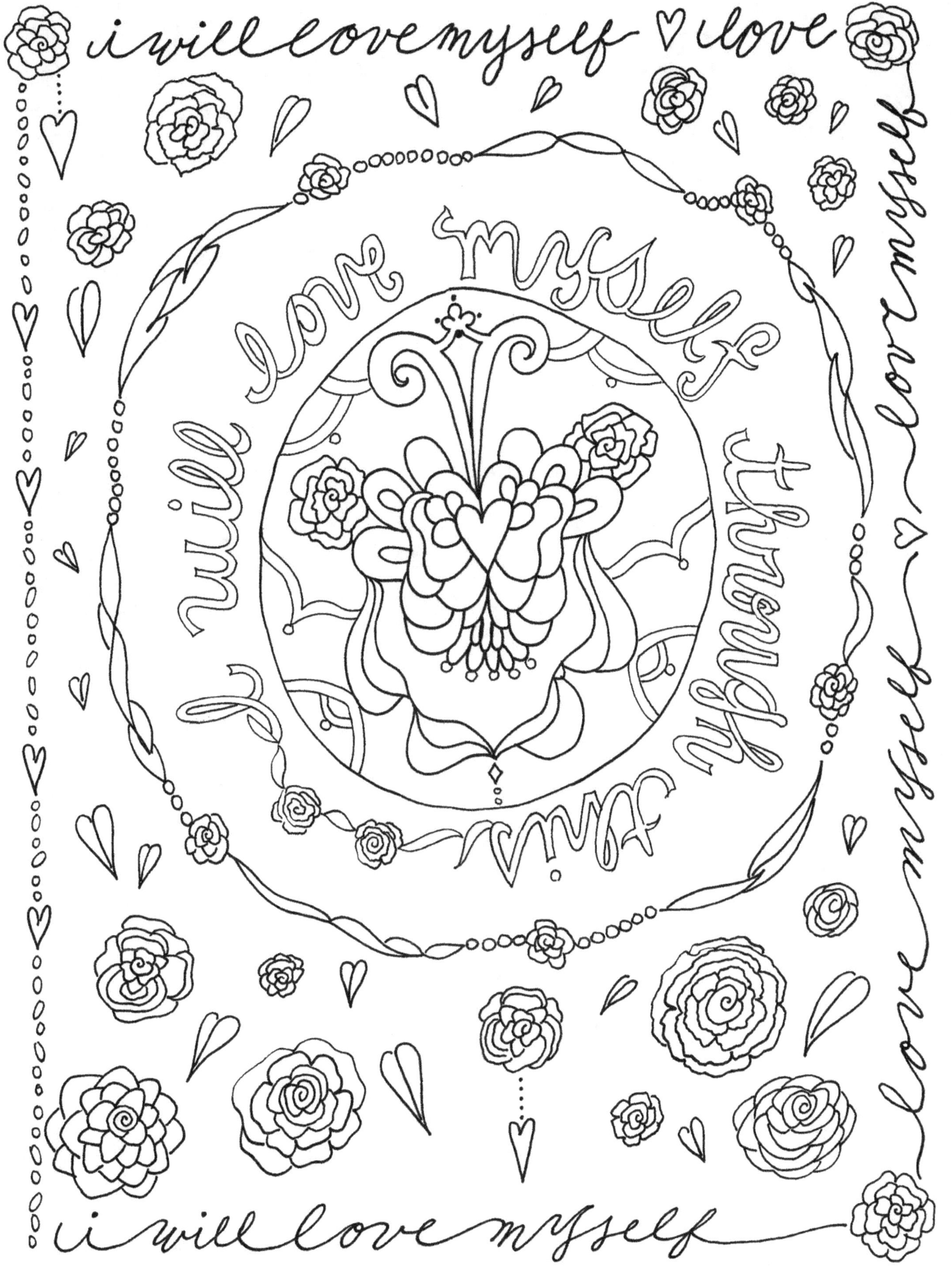
i will love myself ♥ love
love myself
i will love through this
i will love myself

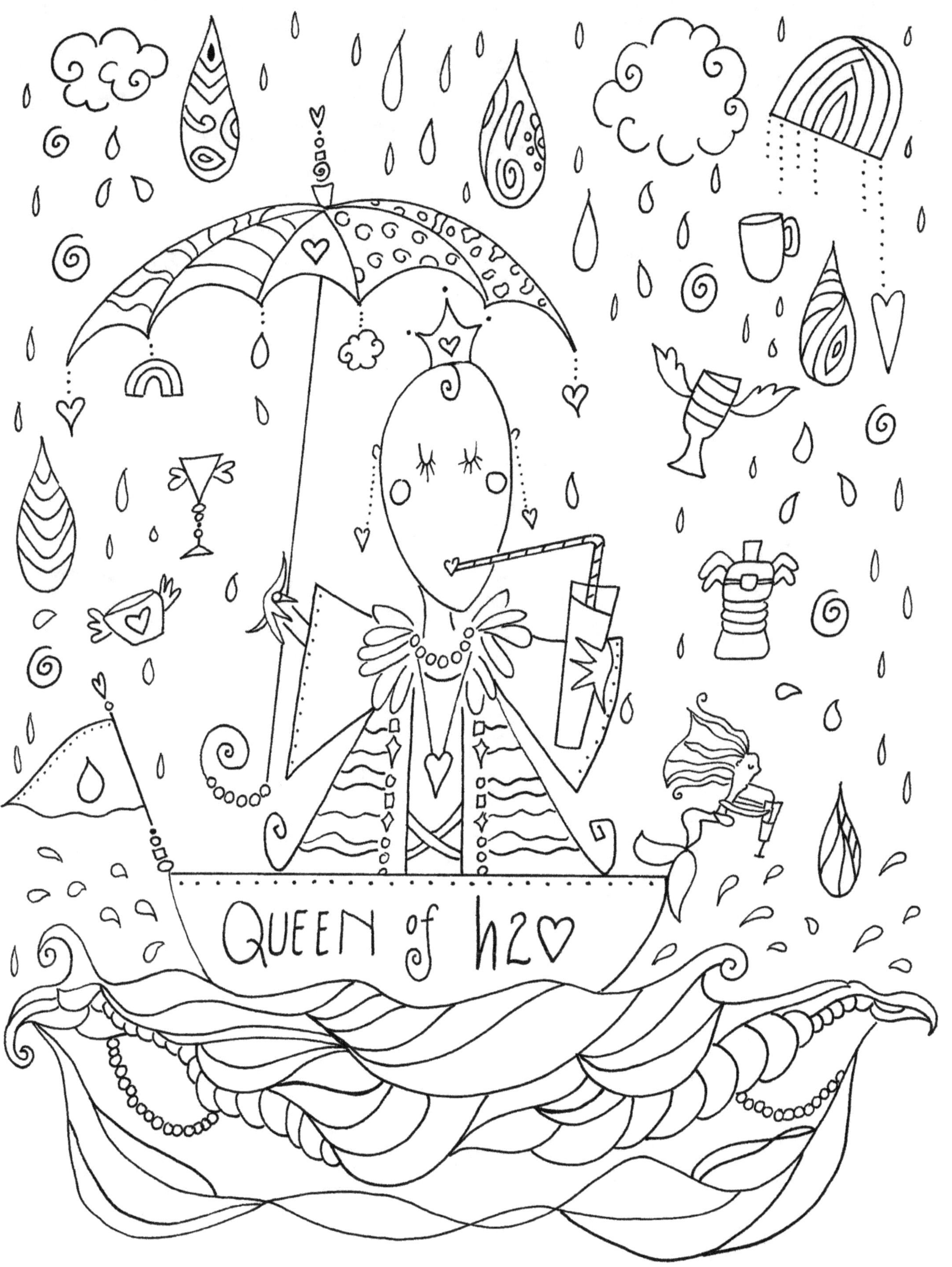

QUEEN of h2♡

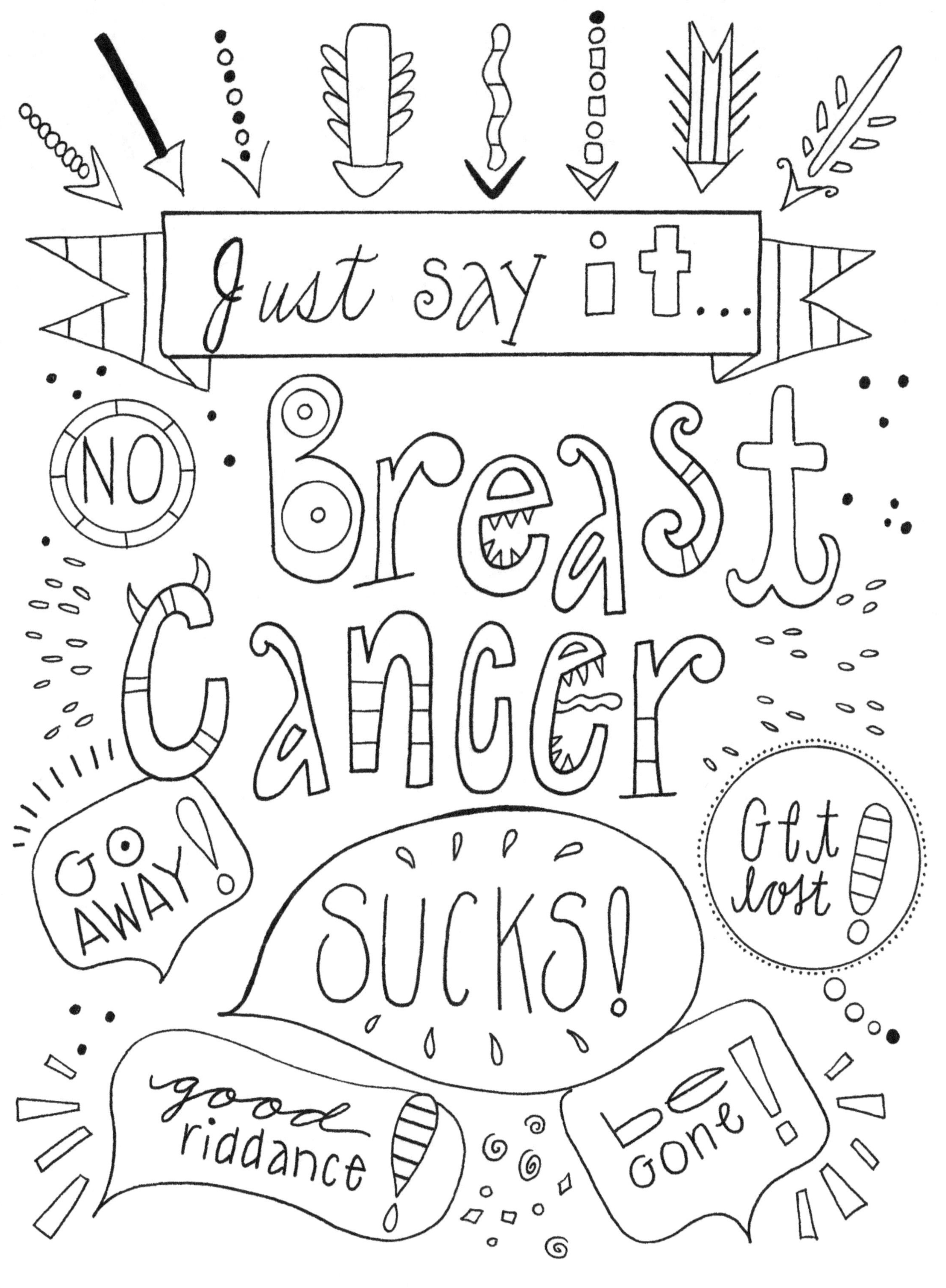

Just say it...
NO Breast Cancer
GO AWAY!
SUCKS!
Get lost!
good riddance
be gone!

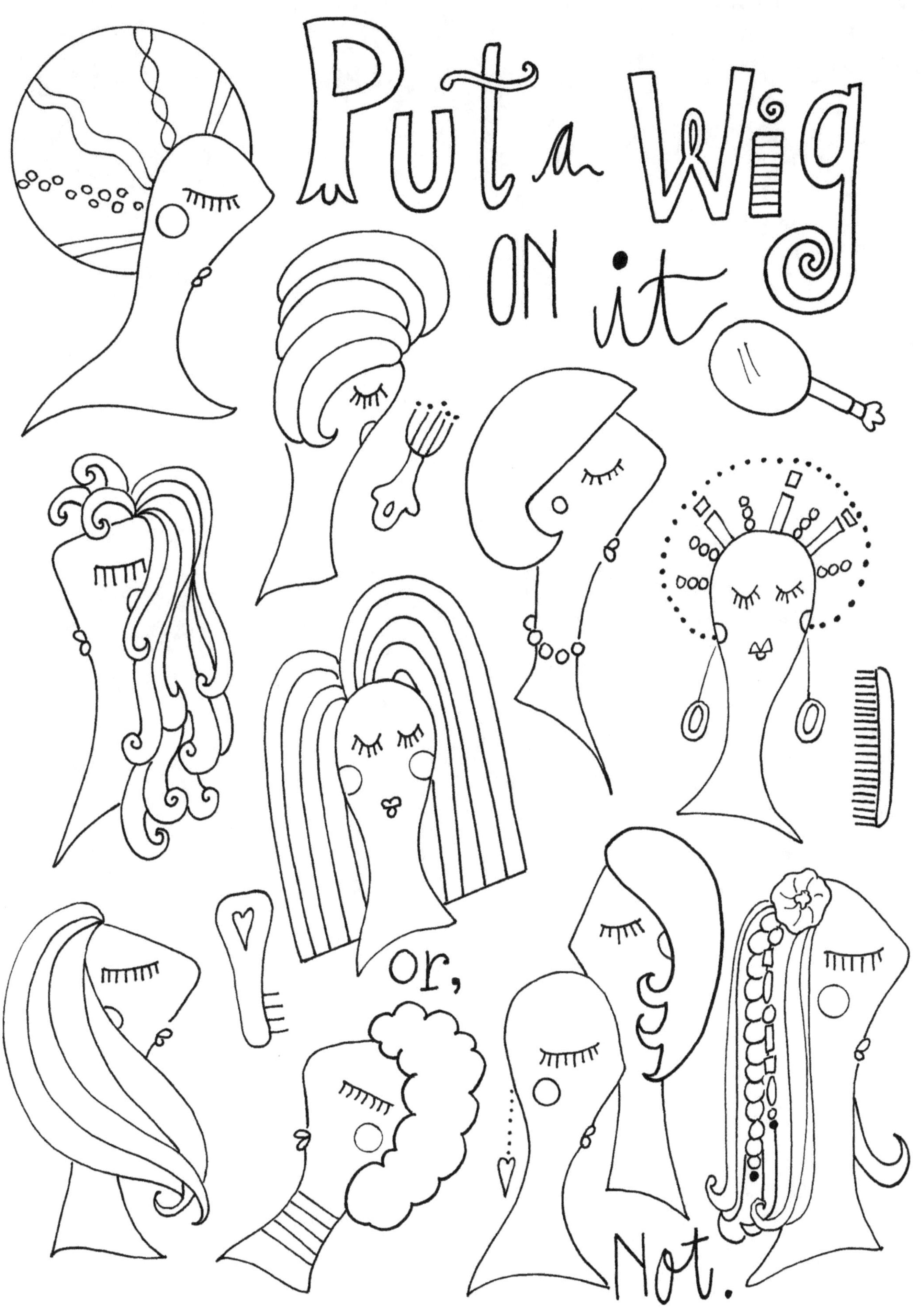
Put a Wig
on it
or,
Not.

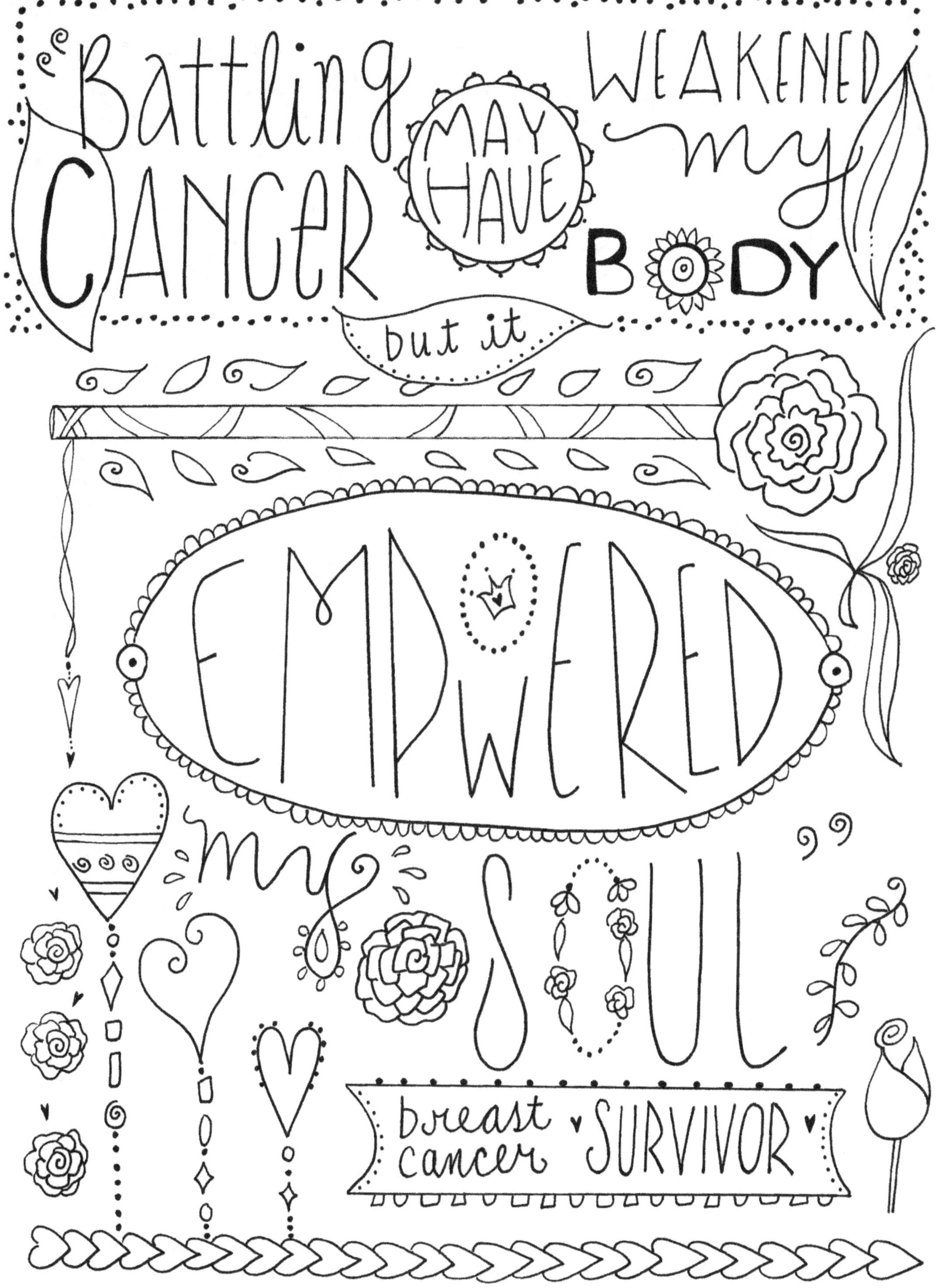

"Battling CANCER MAY HAVE WEAKENED MY BODY but it EMPOWERED my SOUL"
breast cancer SURVIVOR

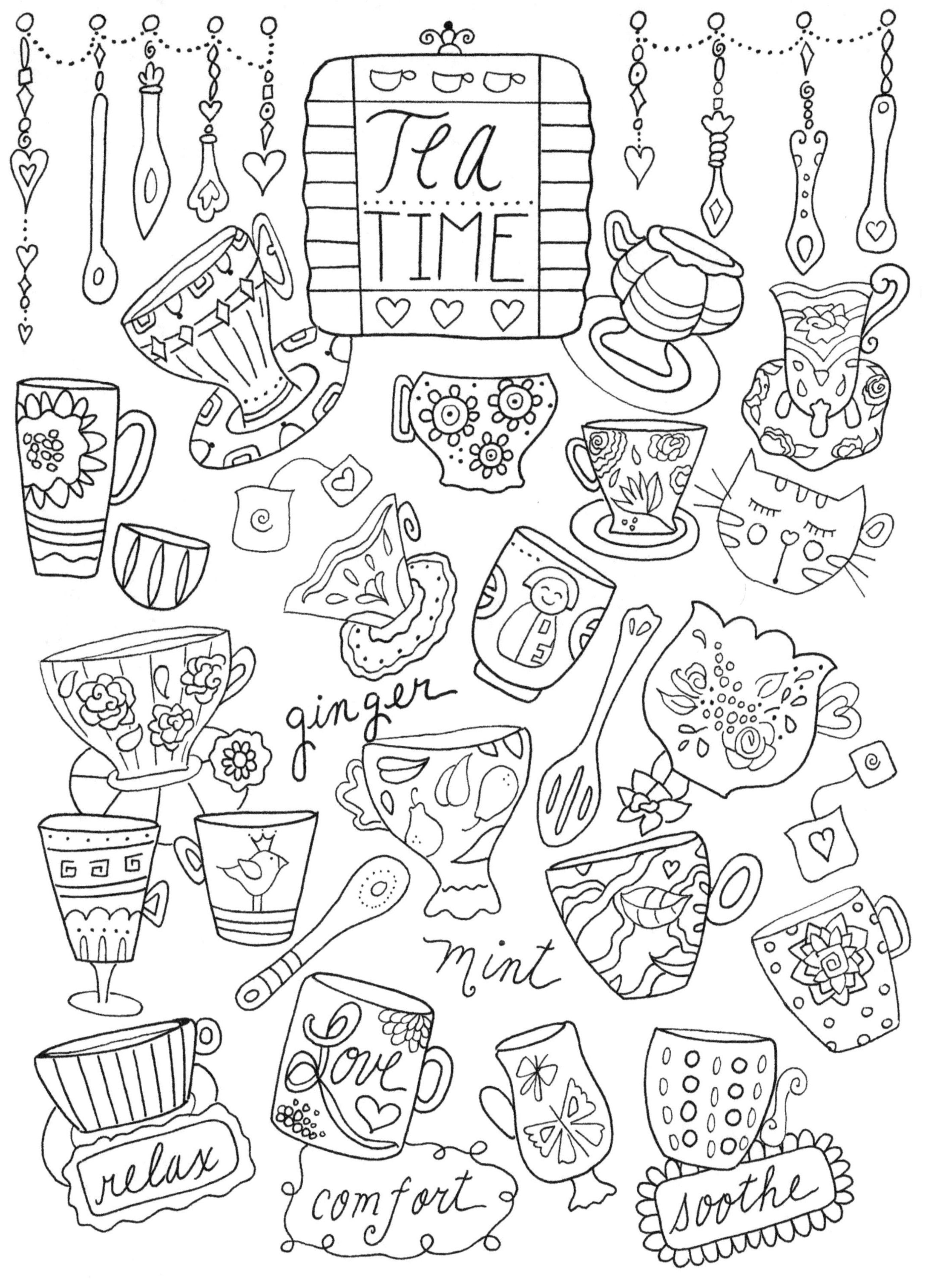

Tea
TIME
ginger
mint
Love
relax
comfort
soothe

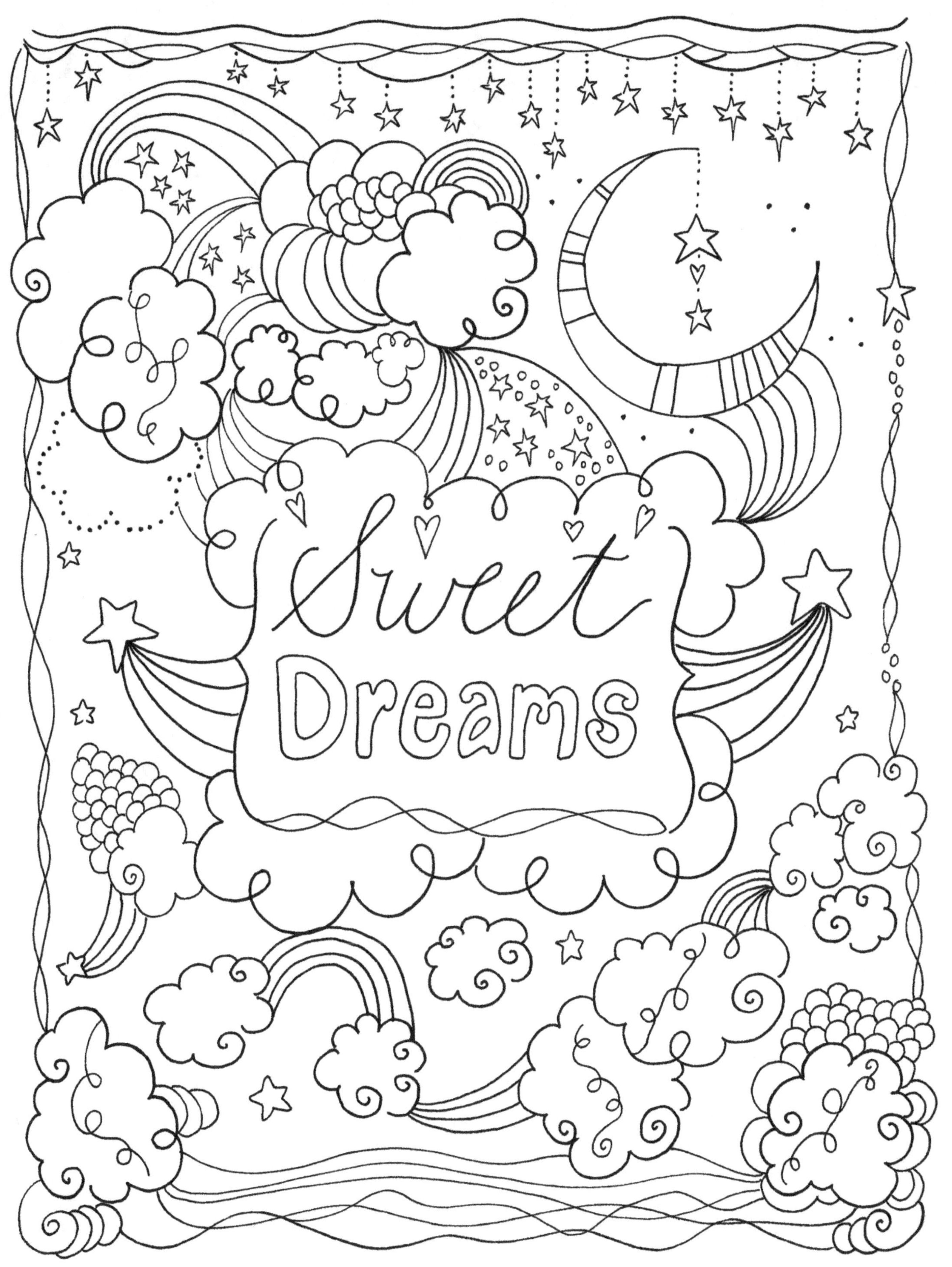

Sweet
Dreams

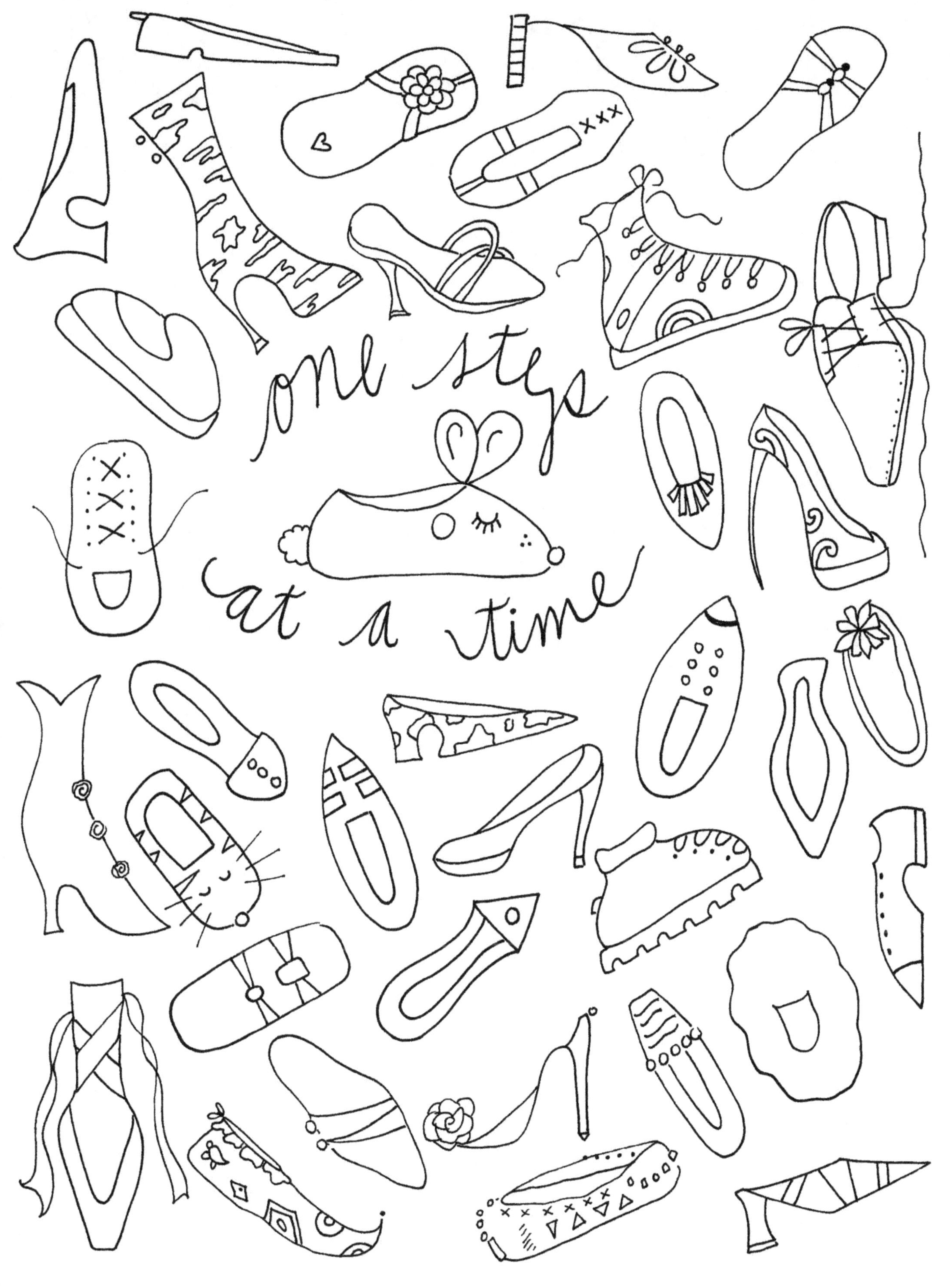
one step
at a time

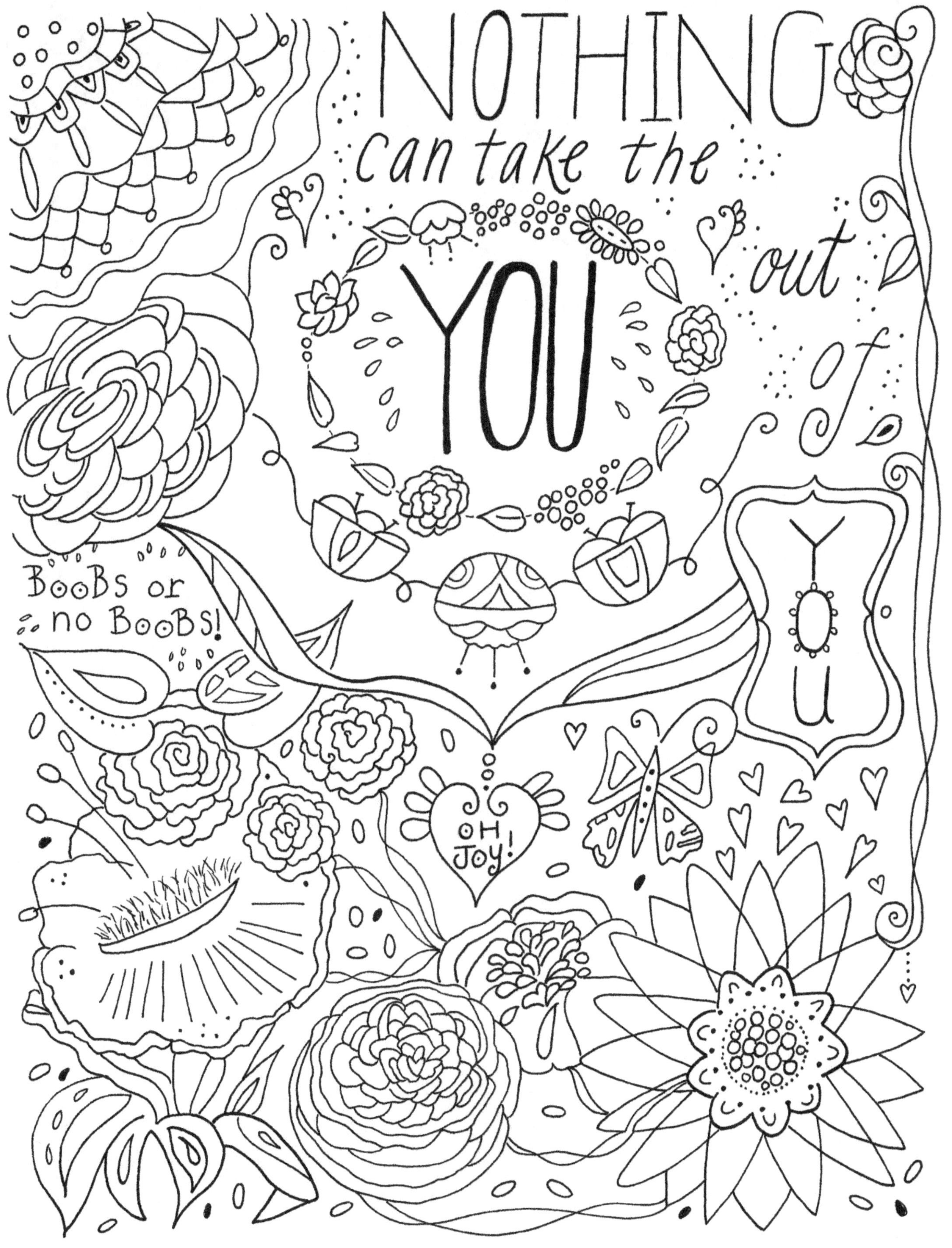

NOTHING
can take the
YOU
out of
YOU
Boobs or no Boobs!
OH JOY!

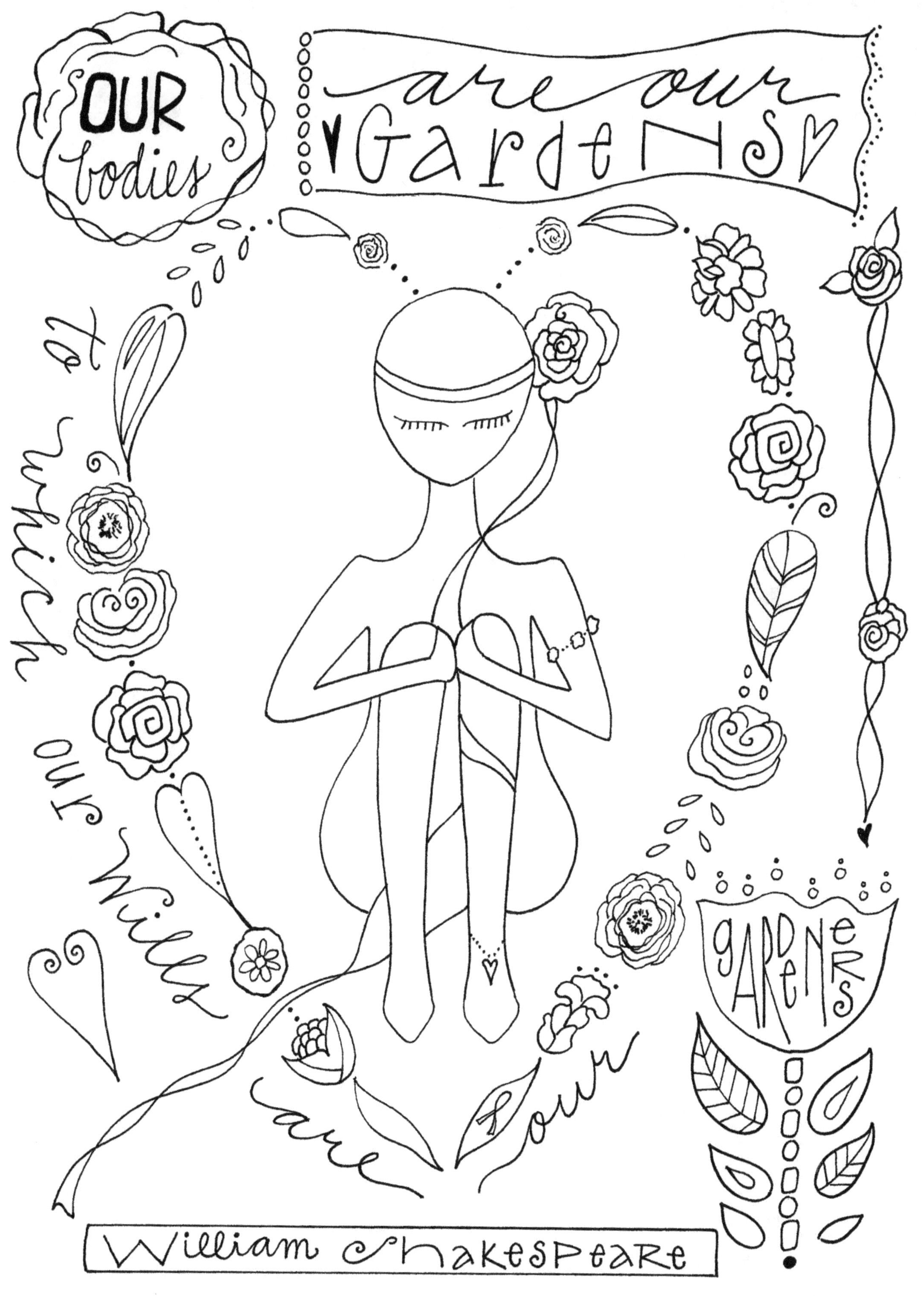

OUR bodies
are our GARDENS
to which our wills
are gardeners
William Shakespeare

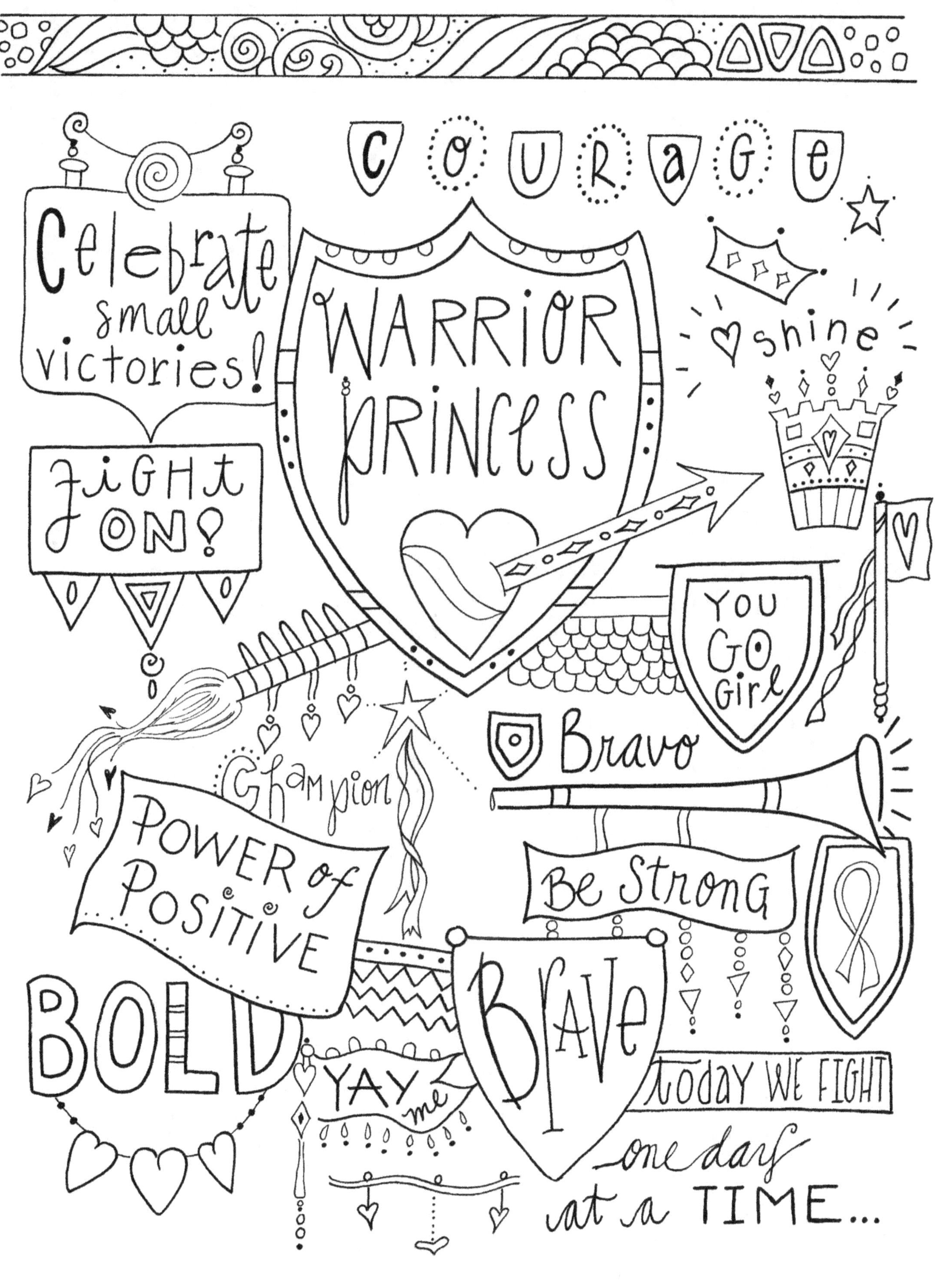

COURAGE
Celebrate small victories!
Fight on!
WARRIOR Princess
shine
You GO Girl
Champion
Bravo
POWER of POSITIVE
Be Strong
BOLD
YAY me
BRAVE
TODAY WE FIGHT
one day at a TIME...

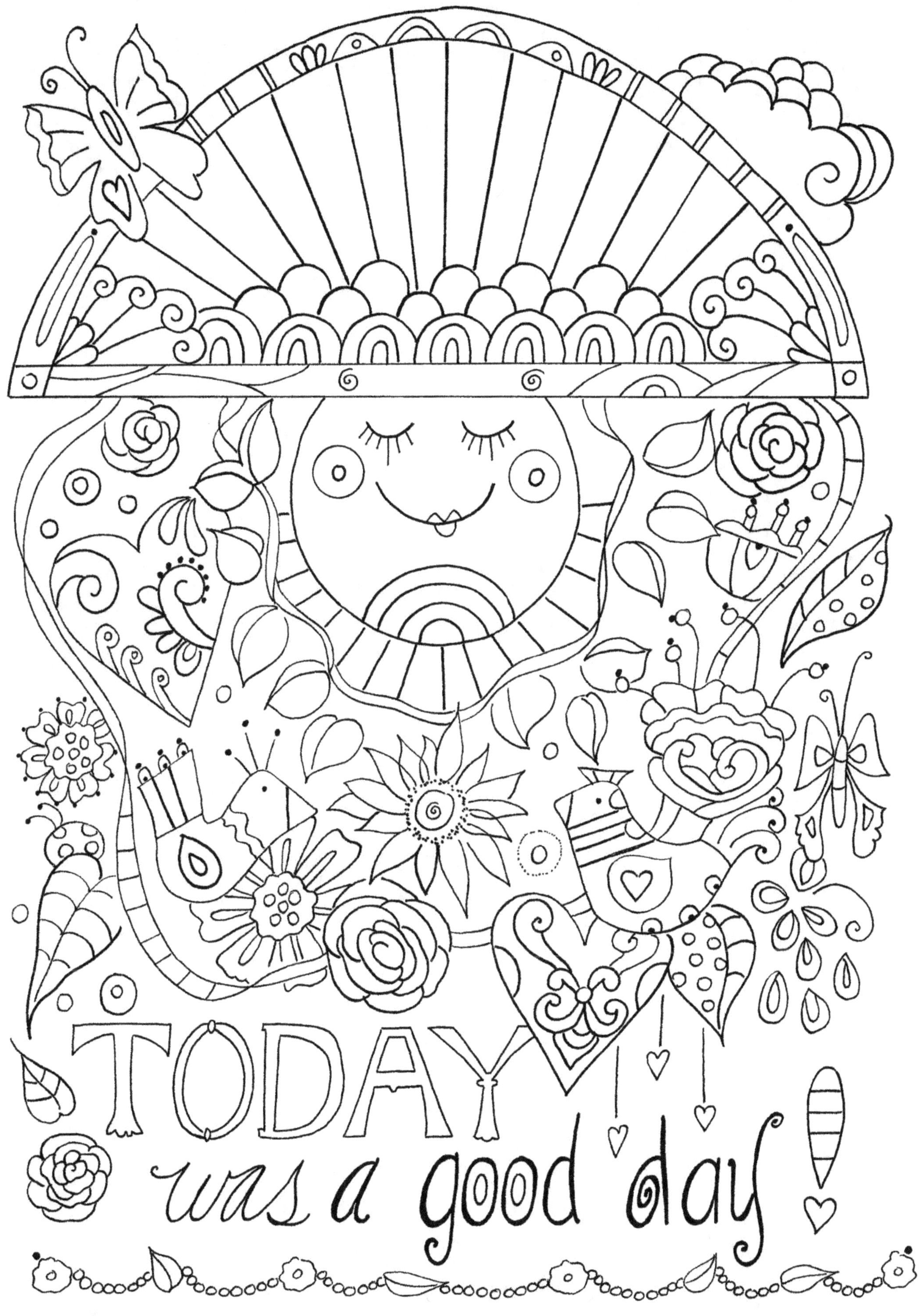

TODAY
was a good day!

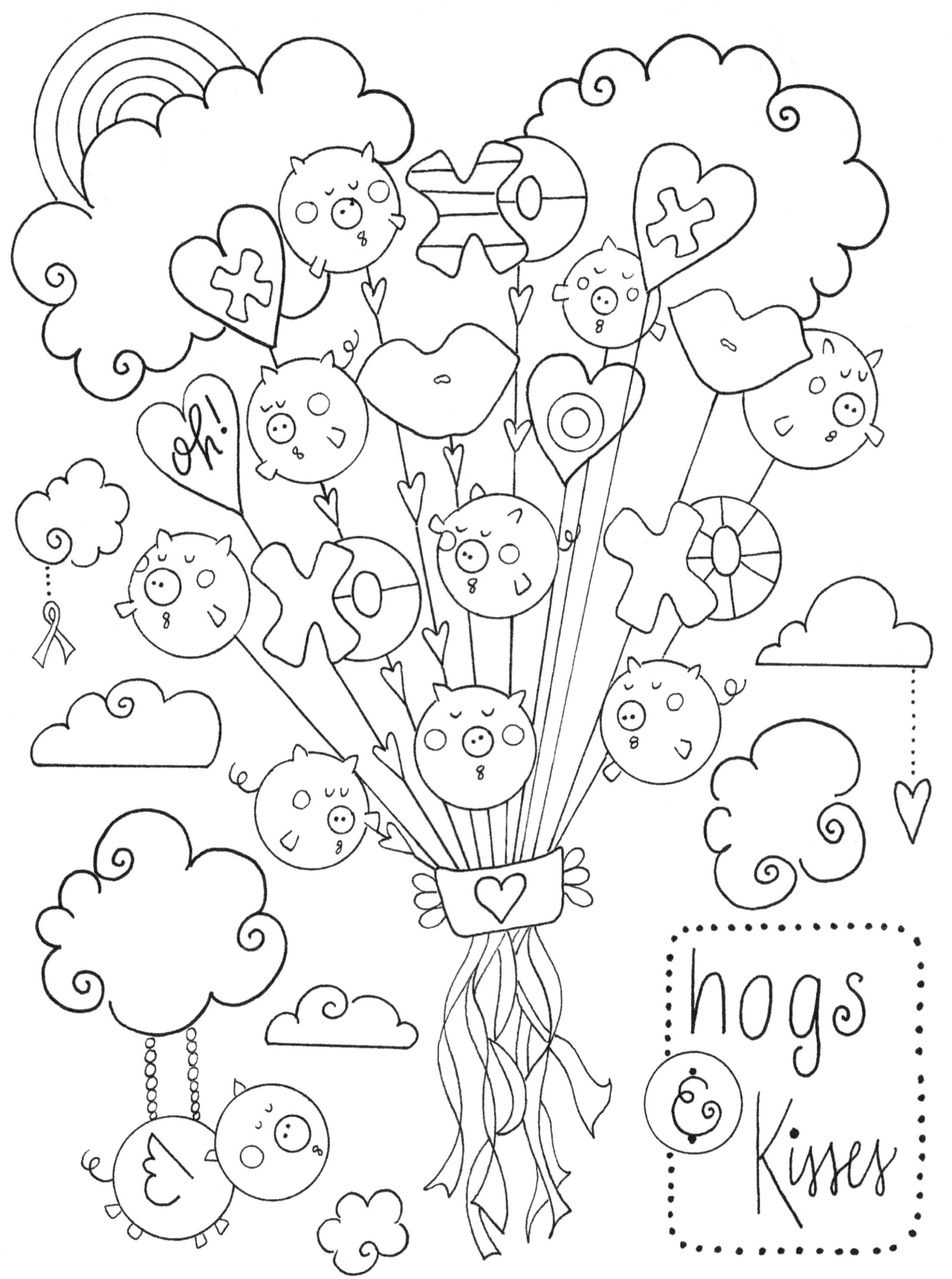

XOXO
oh!
XOXO
XOXO
hogs
&
kisses

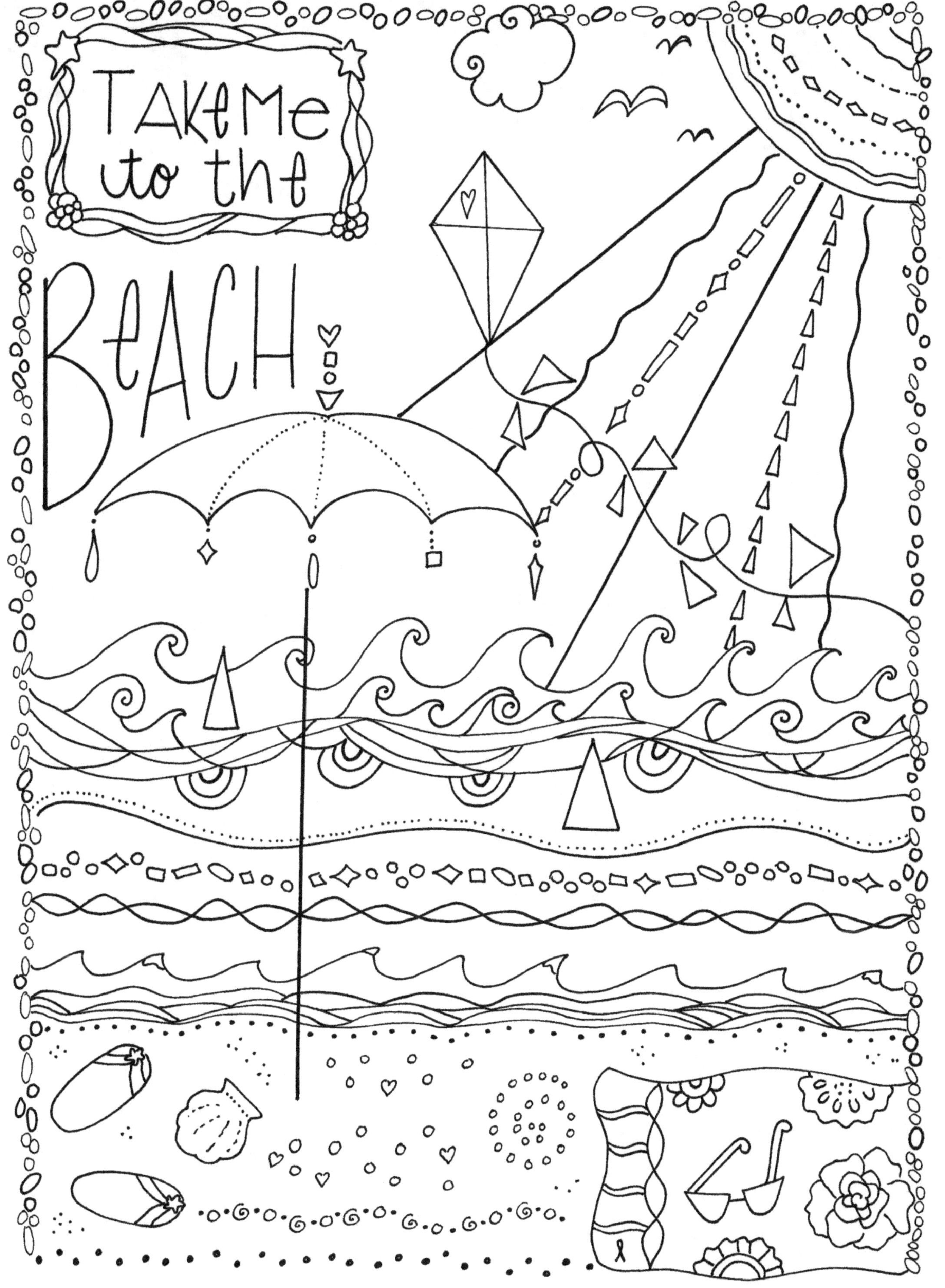

Take Me
to the
BEACH

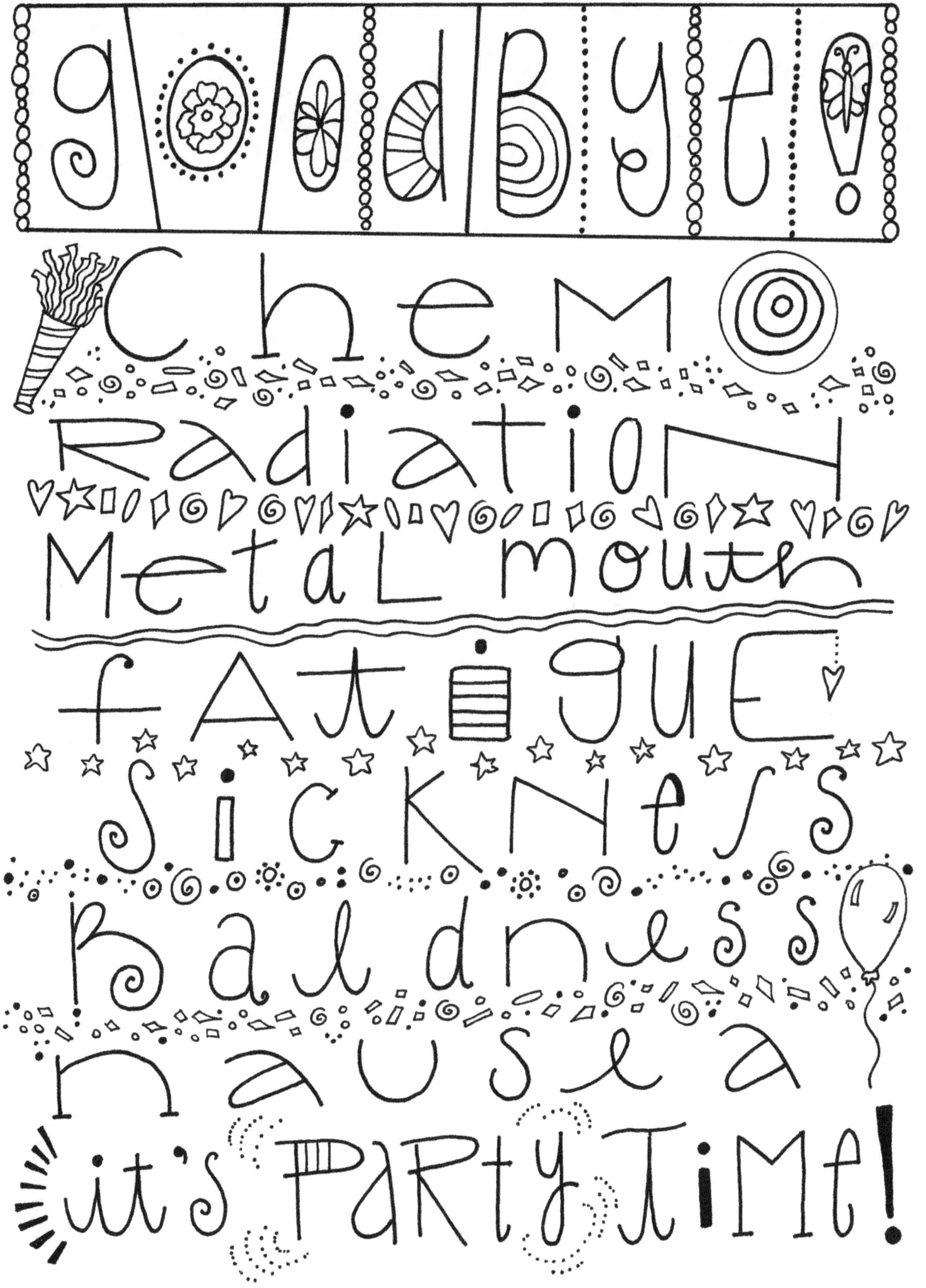

goodbye!
chemo
radiation
metal mouth
fatigue
sickness
baldness
nausea
it's party time!

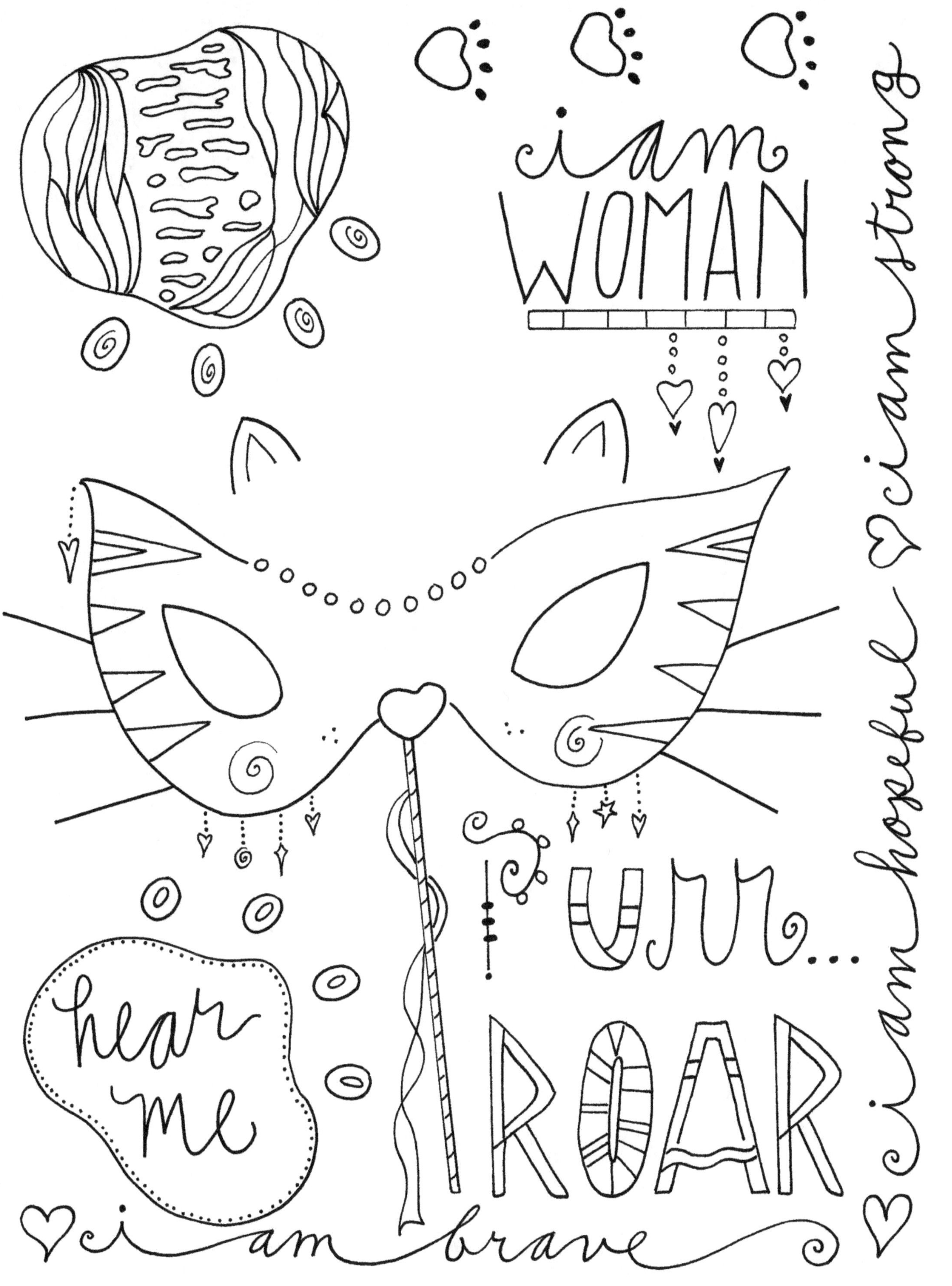
i am
WOMAN
hear
me
PURR...
ROAR
i am brave
i am hopeful
i am strong

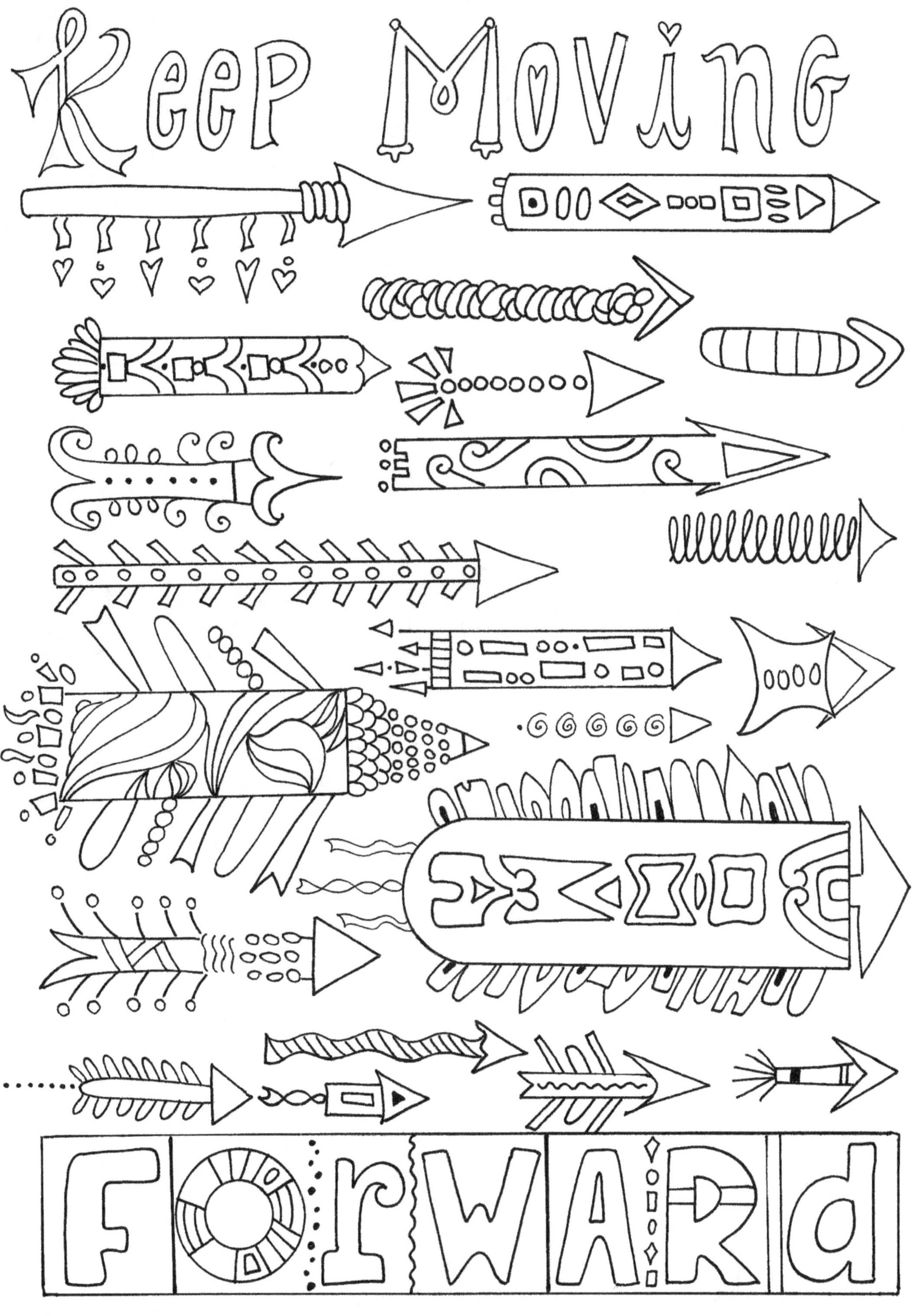

Keep Moving
Forward

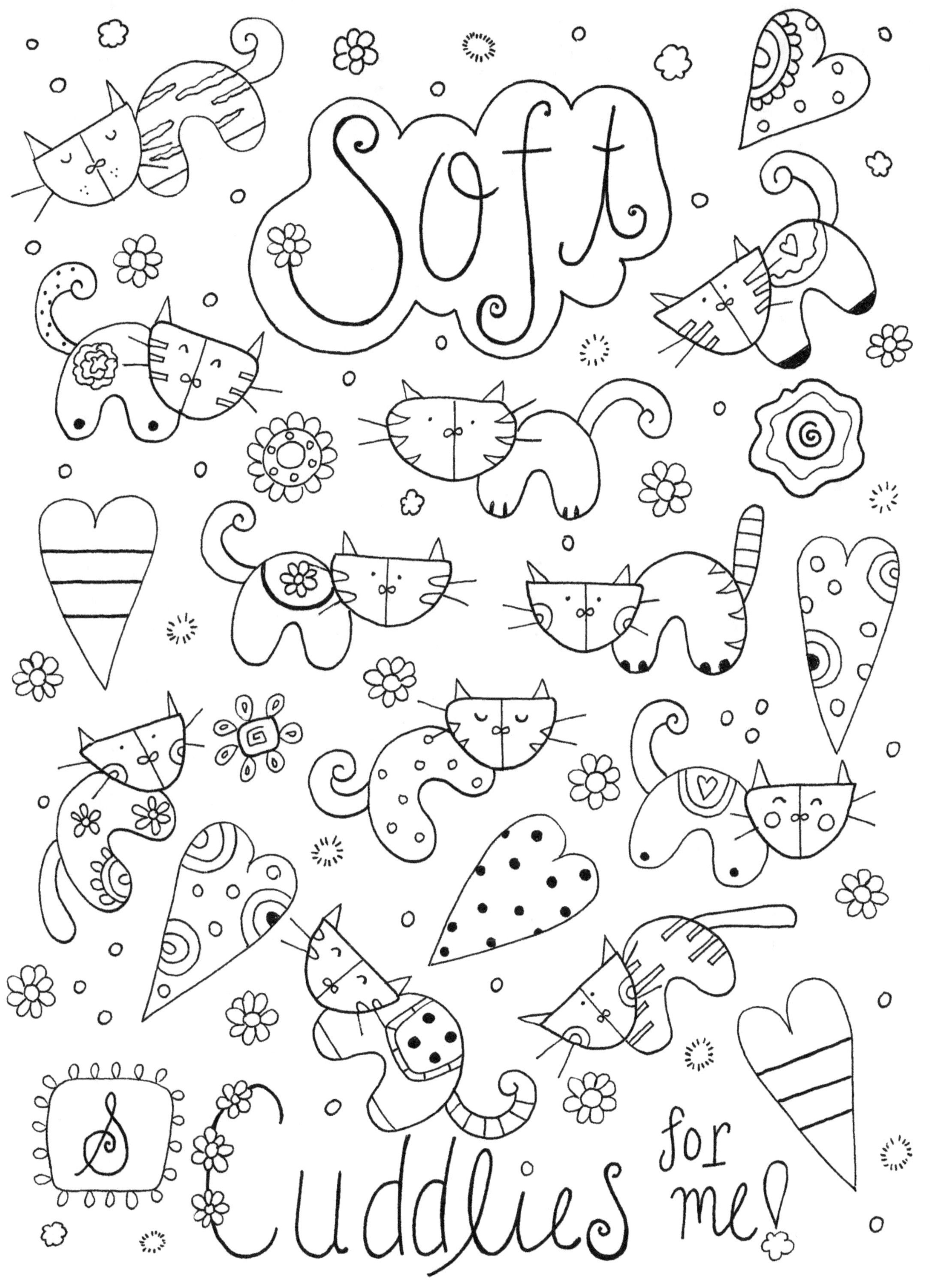

Soft
Cuddlies for me!

She WROTE *her* *her* love LOVE love on her scars

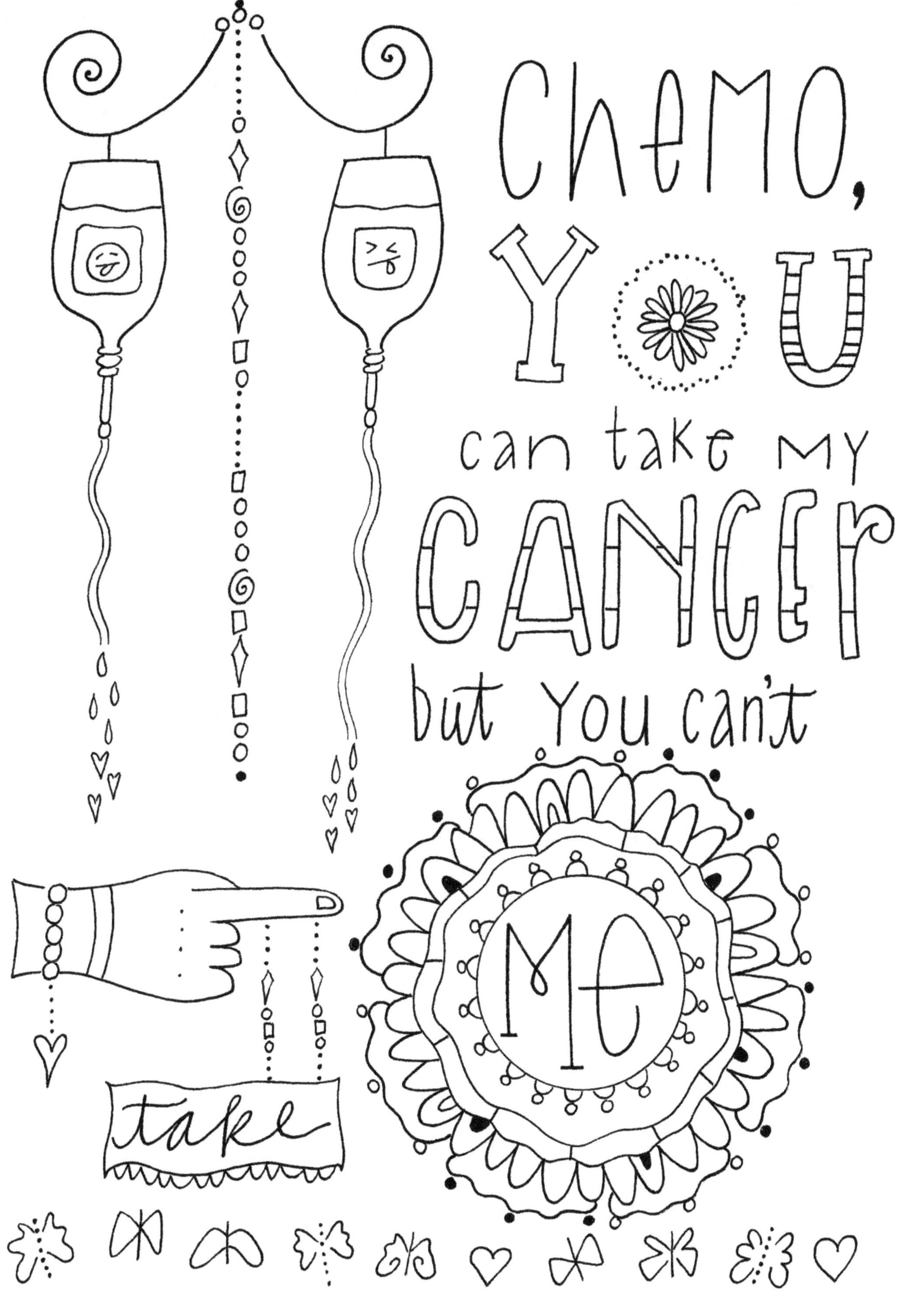

CHEMO, YOU
can take my
CANCER
but you can't
take
ME

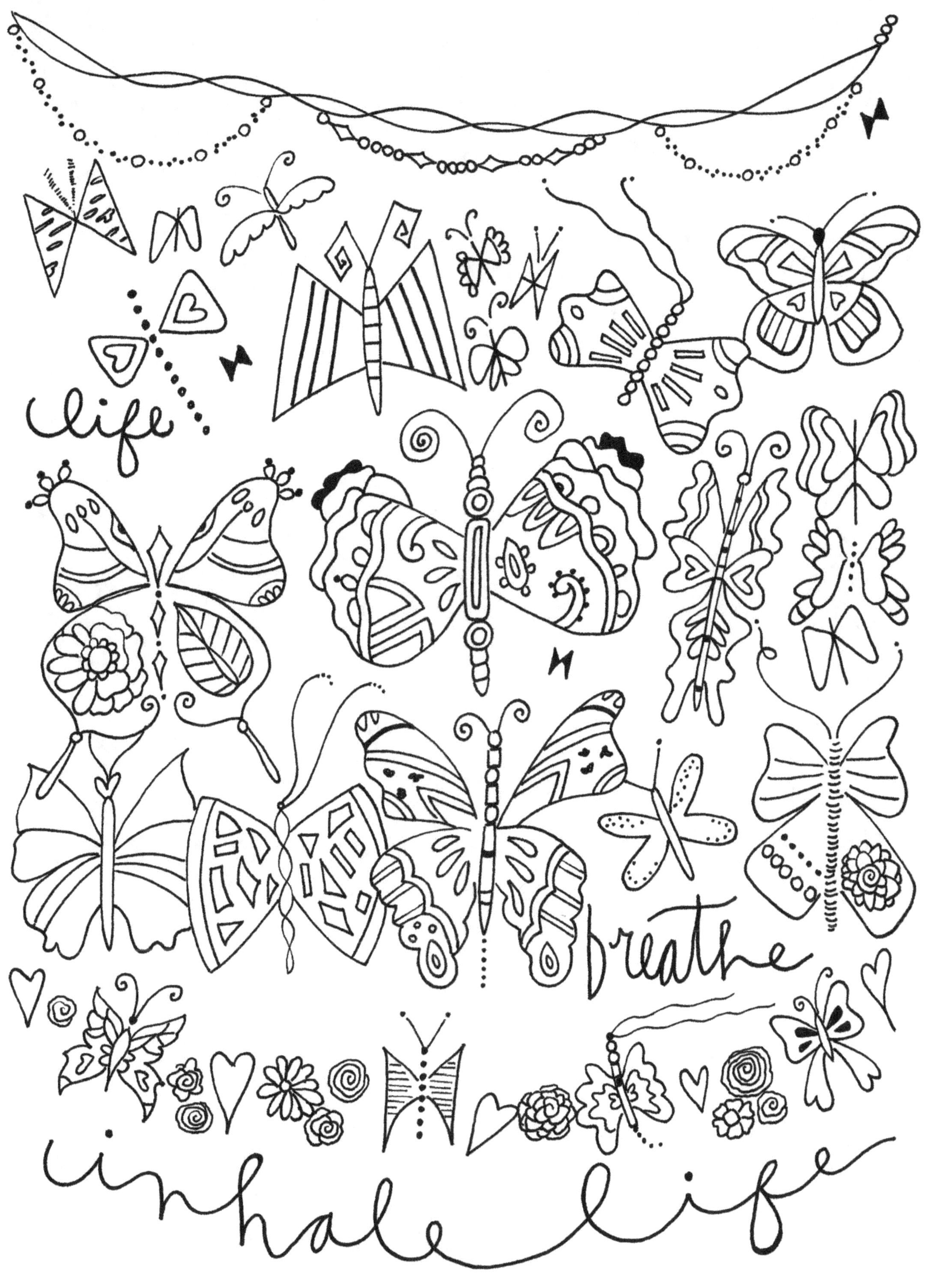
life
breathe
inhale life

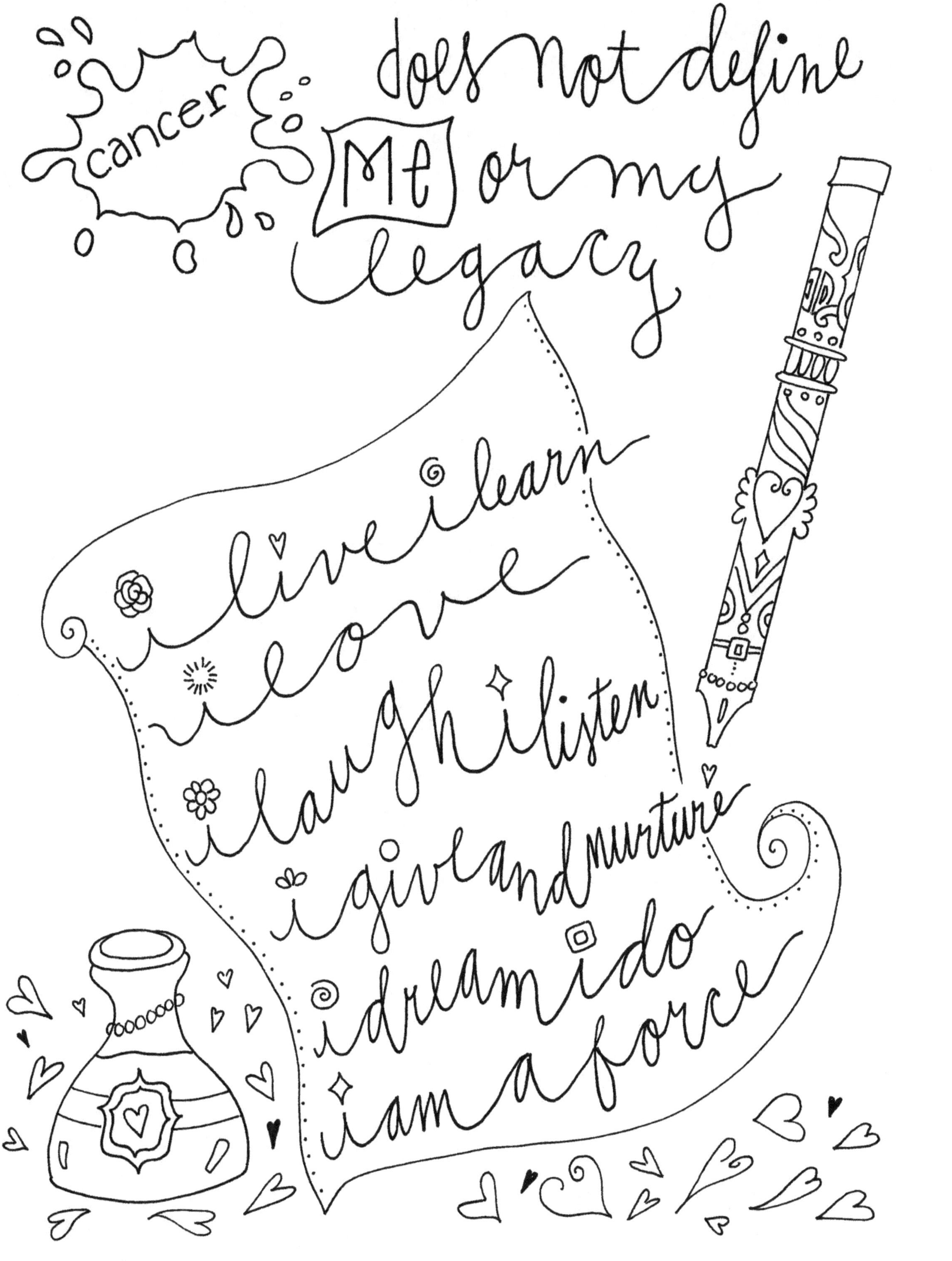

cancer does not define ME or my legacy

i live i learn
i love
i laugh i listen
i give and nurture
i dream i do
i am a force

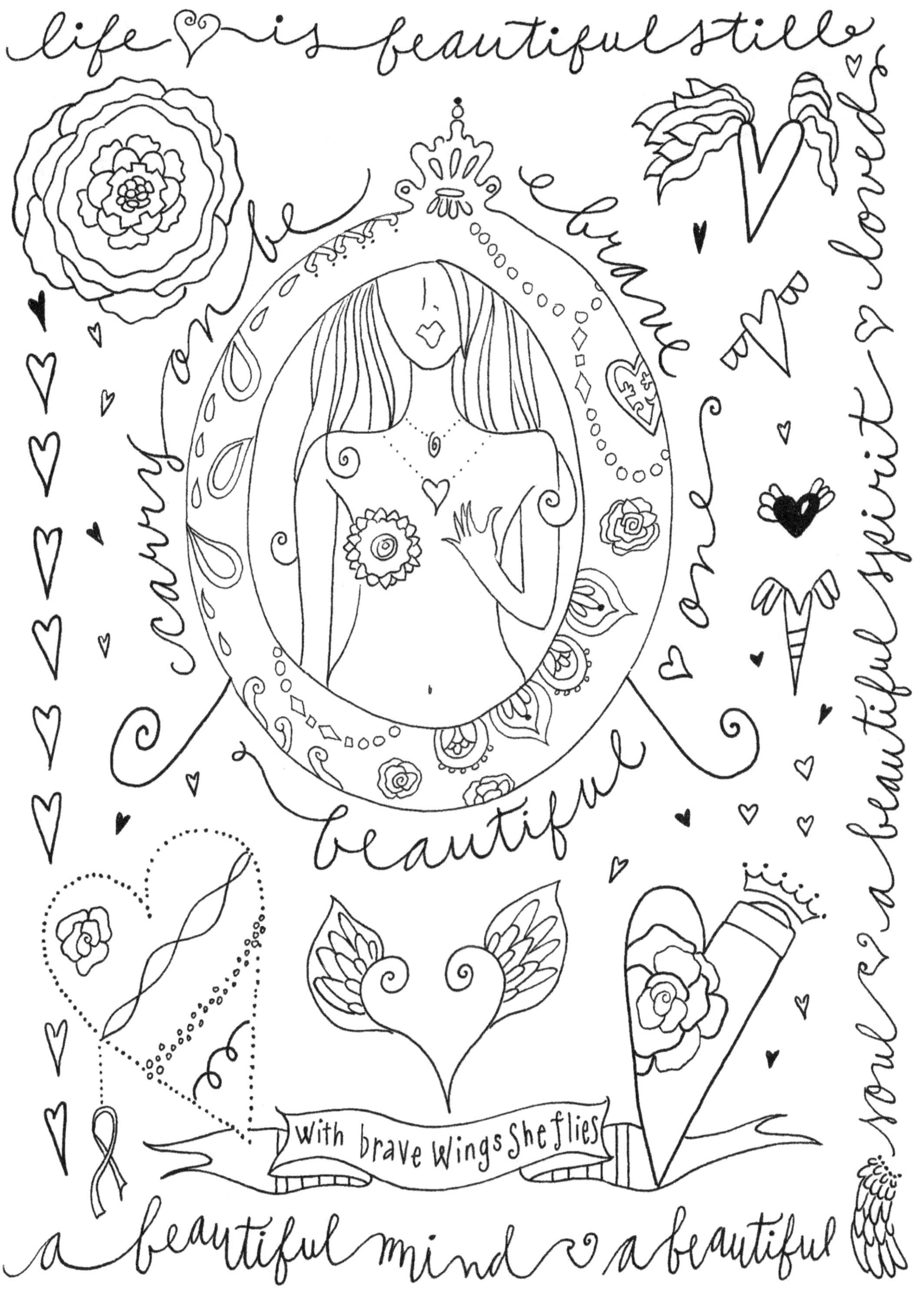

life is beautiful still
carry on be brave
beautiful one
beautiful
with brave wings she flies
a beautiful mind a beautiful
soul a beautiful spirit loved

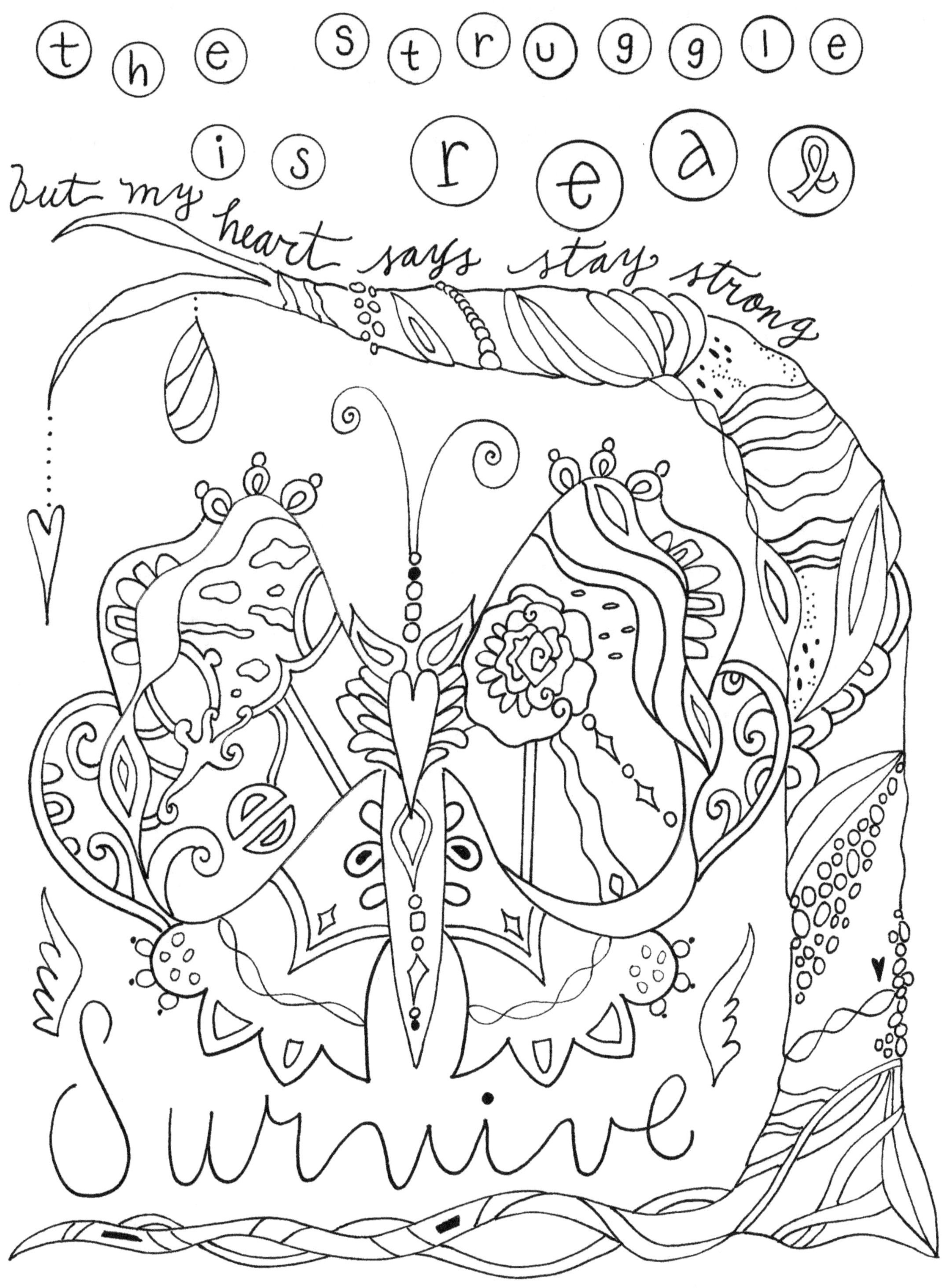

the struggle
is real
but my heart says stay strong
Survive

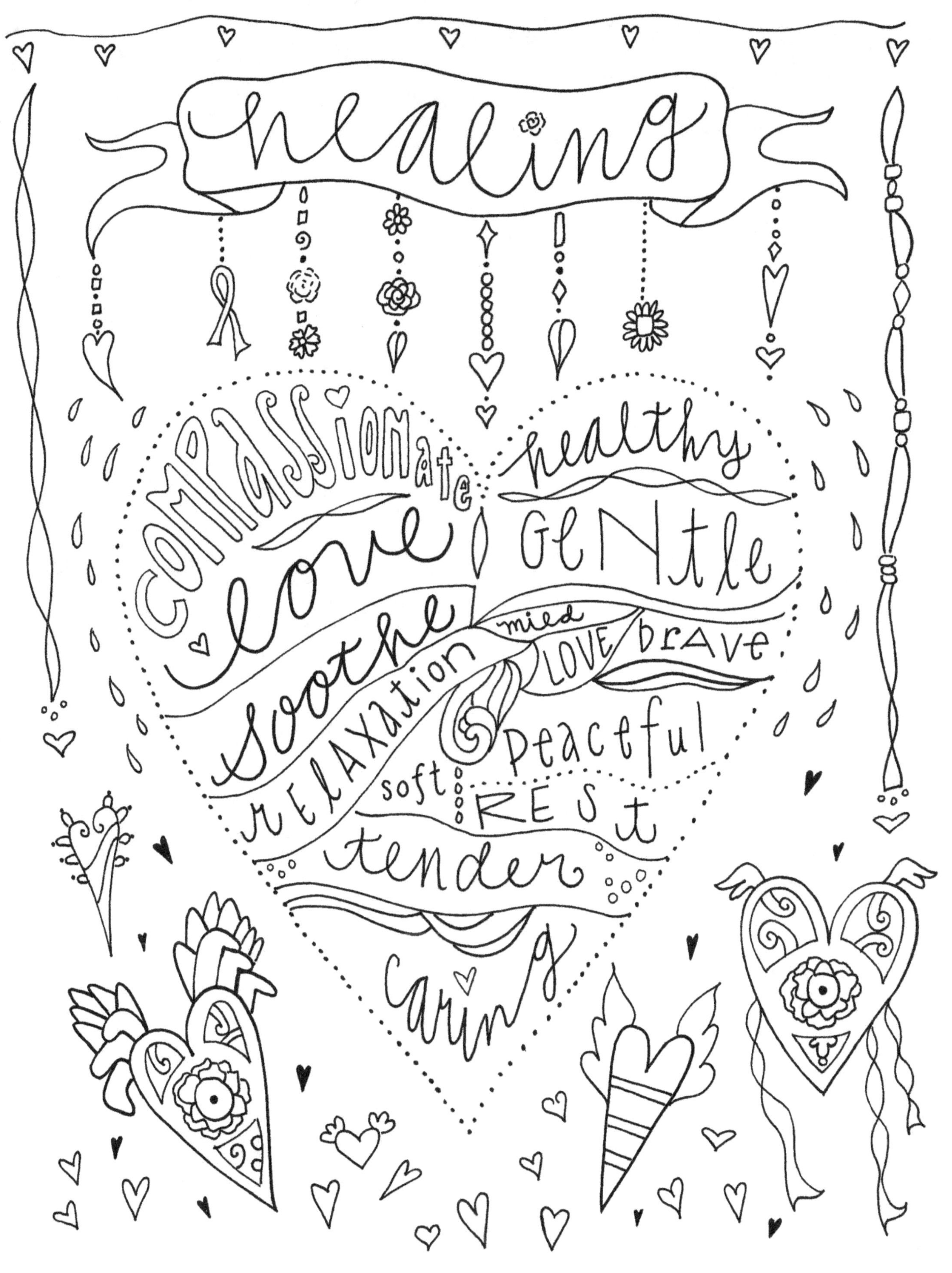

healing
compassionate
love
healthy
gentle
soothe
relaxation
mind
love brave
soft
peaceful
rest
tender
caring

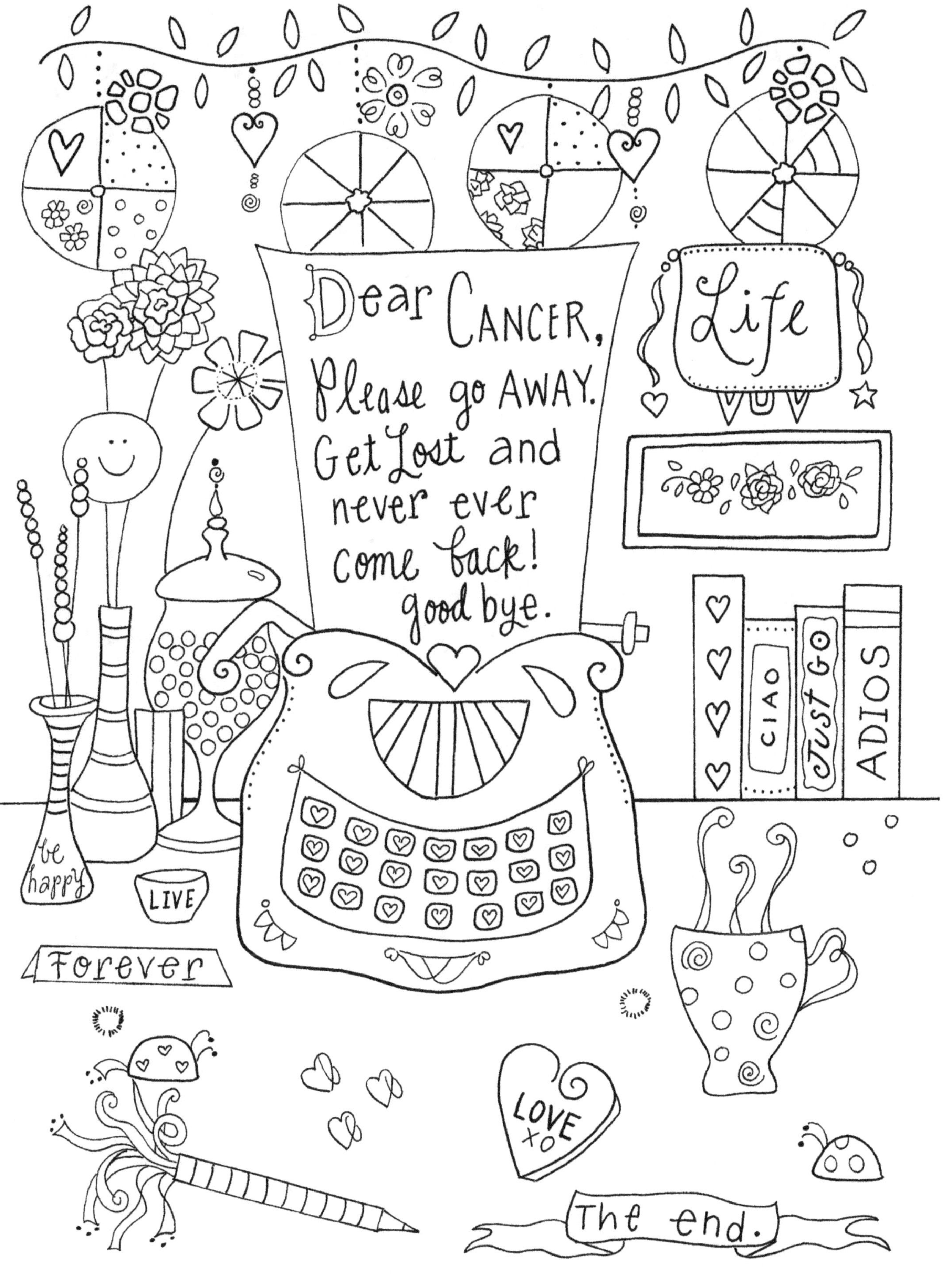

Dear Cancer,
Please go AWAY.
Get Lost and
never ever
come back!
good bye.
Life
be happy
LIVE
Forever
CIAO
Just Go
ADIOS
LOVE to
The end.

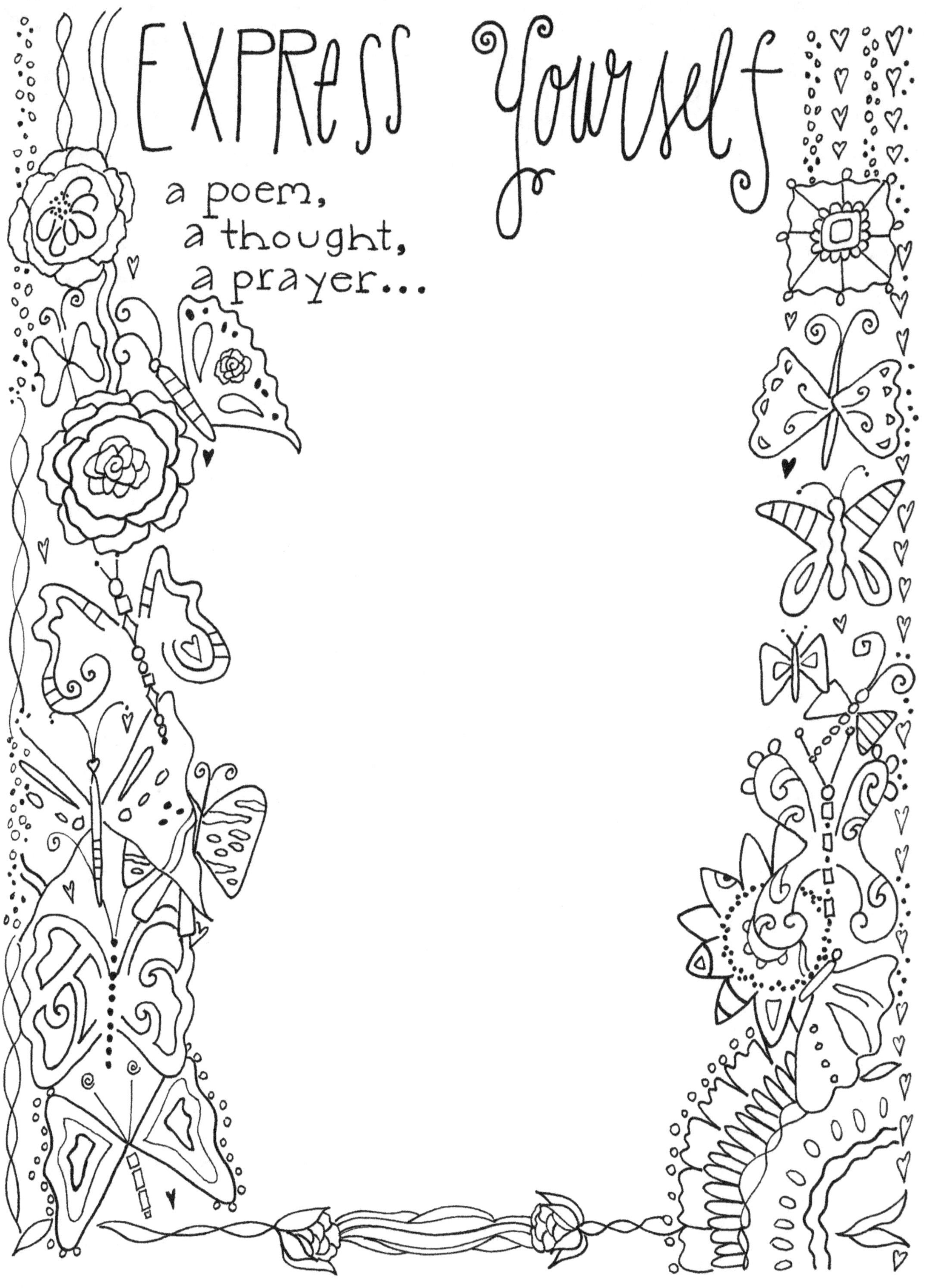

EXPRESS Yourself
a poem,
a thought,
a prayer...

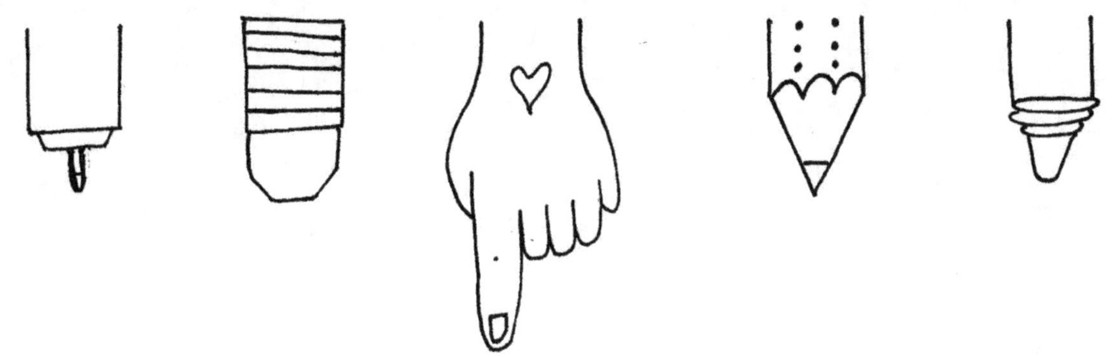

PRACTICE PAGE

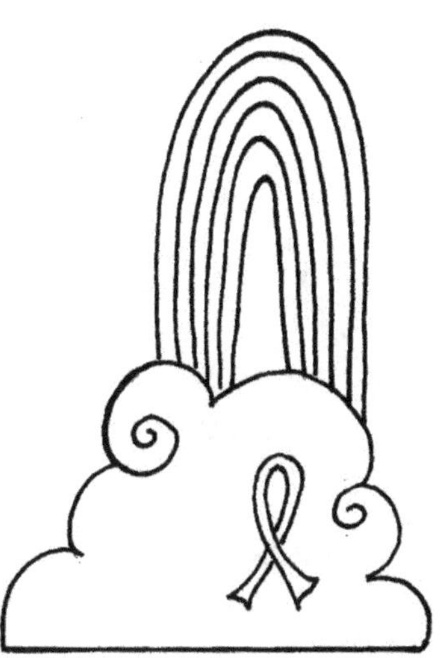

About the Artist...

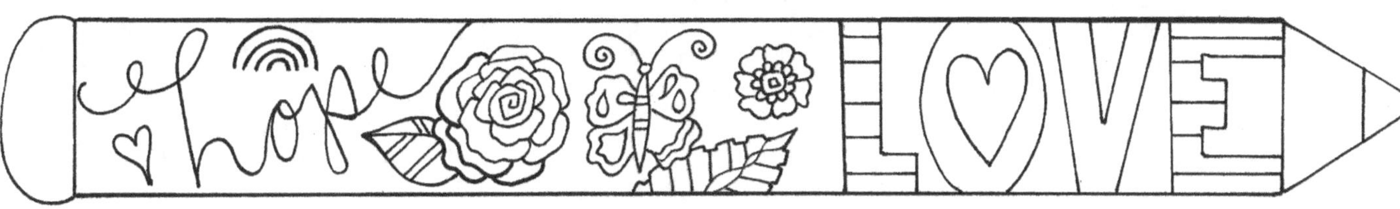

April McCallum is an illustrator, cartoonist and writer. Since retiring from a successful career in the high-tech industry, she's focused her creative passions on art, writing and advocacy projects. Her artwork has been licensed for business and non-profits; and printed on a variety of gift products (posters, greeting cards, mugs, and more.) Her writing and artwork have appeared in a variety of magazines, covers, and featured by CNBC. She's also participated in international art exhibits that raise funds for important causes. Her signature style combines words and visuals, color and design. Her writing and illustration work is inspirational, hope-filled and empowering, while her cartoonist side brings a unique twist of humor to the table.

April has long been an "advocacy artist" designing creative pieces that interweave words and visuals to speak to issues close to her heart. Current topics include breast cancer awareness, empowering women, adoption, human trafficking and violence against women.

Pete Berg and April McCallum have been creative collaborators on a variety of colorful and interesting projects over the years. If you would like to connect with Pete regarding a graphic art project, he can be reached at: ohberg3@gmail.com.

Website:	www.aprilmccallumdesigns.com
Email:	april@aprilmccallumdesigns.com
Facebook:	@AprilMcCallumDesigns
Instagram:	@AprilCartoons | @PinkCartoons
Twitter:	@AprilCartoons | @PinkCartoons
Pinterest:	https://www.pinterest.com/aprilmccallum/
	https://www.pinterest.com/pinkpassionlife/

www.ingramcontent.com/pod-product-compliance
Lightning Source LLC
Chambersburg PA
CBHW081624250726
48657CB00009B/2716